IMPERIAL MEDICINE

IMPERIAL MEDICINE

*Patrick Manson and the
Conquest of Tropical Disease*

DOUGLAS M. HAYNES

PENN

UNIVERSITY OF PENNSYLVANIA PRESS

Philadelphia

10 9 8 7 6 5 4 3 2 1

Published by
University of Pennsylvania Press
Philadelphia, Pennsylvania 19104–4011

Library of Congress Cataloging-in-Publication Data
Haynes, Douglas Melvin.
   Imperial medicine : Patrick Manson and the conquest of tropical
disease / by Douglas M. Haynes.
      p. ; cm.
   Includes bibliographical references and index.
   ISBN 0-8122-3598-3 (cloth : alk. paper)
      1. Manson, Patrick, Sir, 1844–1922.   2. Tropical medicine—
Great Britain—History.   3. Physicians—Great Britain—Biography.
I. Title.
[DNLM: 1. Manson, Patrick, Sir, 1844–1922.   2. Tropical
Medicine—history.   3. Colonialism—history.   4. History of Medicine,
19th Cent.   5. Malaria—history.   6. Tropical Medicine—Biography.
WZ 100 M2897H 2001]
RC962.G7 H39   2001
616.9'883'092—dc21
[B]   00-068268

Contents

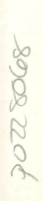

Illustrations and Tables

Introduction
British Medicine as Imperial Medicine

THIS book is about the role of British imperialism in the making of Victorian medicine and science. The career of Patrick Manson, the "father" of the modern study of tropical medicine, serves as the point of departure for an exploration of this relationship from the mid-nineteenth century until the early twentieth century. Why Manson? He is worthy of a book-length study not least because of his pioneering research into the role of the mosquito in the development and spread of the *Plasmodia* protozoa (the cause of malaria disease) and other human pathogens. As medical adviser to the Colonial Office (1895–1911), Manson also played a critical role in the domestication of research into the diseases of the tropical empire at the London School of Tropical Medicine, which was founded in 1898 and continues to operate. Moreover, in the wake of decolonization, Manson's reputation has provided a contested ground for specialists and historians alike who are engaged in forging an understanding of the place of Western medicine and science in European imperialism and its lingering consequences.

This study is by no means the first. There have been two earlier biographies of Manson. The first, coauthored by Col. Alfred Alcock and P. H. Manson-Bahr (Manson's son-in-law and later research protégé), appeared in 1927, some five years after Manson's death. In 1962, Manson-Bahr was the sole author of *Patrick Manson: Father of Tropical Medicine*.[1] Each biography reflects the affection of Manson-Bahr and Alcock for Manson based on their long professional association and personal ties. As patron, Manson was instrumental in the appointment of Alcock, a retired member of the Indian Medical Service, to the London School as medical entomologist in 1905, where he remained a fixture for over a decade.[2] Manson-Bahr married Manson's daughter Edith Margaret in 1909 and in 1921 assumed the editorship of the textbook *Tropical Disease*, which Manson first published in 1898.[3] After Manson died in 1922, Manson-Bahr became his most devoted memorialist. In articles, addresses, and books, he singlehandedly established Manson's reputation as the founder of tropical medicine.[4]

Manson's reputation is not simply a product of the intersection of personal and professional relationships. More important, it forms a discursive site for locating the place of British medicine and science in society and the wider world. As a self-made man from a commercial family in Aberdeenshire, Scotland, Manson had a career that epitomized the openness of medicine and affirmed the "lad of parts" national myth in which social mobility was the reward for the ambitious and resourceful aspirants of the middle and upper classes.[5] After receiving his medical degree at Aberdeen University in 1866, Manson yielded to "an urge to travel" or "adventurous spirit" and launched his career as a port surgeon for the Imperial Chinese Customs Service.[6] For Manson-Bahr, this impulse provided a fortuitous opportunity for the diffusion of western medicine. Over nearly twenty-five years, Manson's effectiveness as a surgeon and practitioner among the inhabitants of south China enriched him while confirming the superiority of Western medicine as a system of healing.[7] Indeed, the College of Medicine of Hong Kong, which Manson helped found in 1887, continued the process of modernizing China by training future generations of practitioners in Western medicine long after he had returned to Britain in 1889.[8]

Manson's reputation derives in large part from his scientific endeavors in the tropical periphery. Pride of place is given to his 1877 discovery of the role of the mosquito in the development of the *filaria* worm.[9] (The presence of this worm in the human body causes a range of diseases along the lymphatic vessels and extremities chiefly by disrupting the flow of fluids in the body.) The importance of this discovery rests not so much on *filaria* disease—which affected primarily the indigenous inhabitants—as on Manson's later application of the mosquito-parasite relationship to the problem of the transmission of malaria.

In practical and cultural terms, malaria posed the single greatest challenge to the expansion of European colonies. The wide swaths of the tropics, ranging from Africa to South America to China, designated as the "white man's grave" testified to stubbornly high levels of mortality and morbidity among European imperial servants. In defining the boundaries of European civilization, this designation defined its comparative absence as well. Manson's 1894 mosquito-malaria theory turned the tables on the tropical natural world, however. In four years, Manson and his collaborator, Ronald Ross in India, discovered the transmission of the *plasmodia* via the bite of the female mosquito. This milestone of British medical science enabled doctors to combat malaria and thus opened up the tropical world to European civilization.

Mosquito Experiment with Hin-Lo (Figure 1) nicely illustrates the wider cultural significance of Manson's discovery in China. The oil painting depicts his seminal 1877 mosquito-biting experiment in Amoy. Manson isolated the role of the *Culex fatigans* mosquito in the development of the *filaria* by using his Chinese servant Hin-Lo as an experimental subject. With the aid of a mosquito-proof screen, Manson created an experimental space in a crude shed. Hin-Lo, whose blood teemed with *filaria* embryos, lay asleep. By opening the screened door at dusk and closing it at sunrise, Manson allowed wild mosquitoes to enter and feast on his servant's blood. Once satiated, they came to rest on the walls of the shed. Over a six-day period, Manson's other servant plucked these mosquitoes and stored them in glass containers. With the aid of a microscope, over

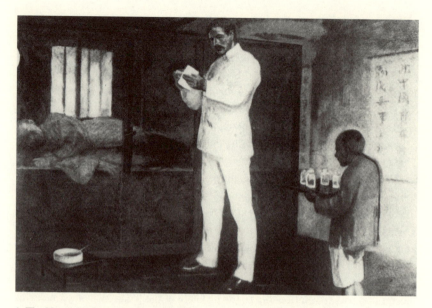

1. *The Mosquito Experiment with Hin-Lo*. From Philip H. Manson-Bahr, *Patrick Manson: The Father of Tropical Medicine* (London: Thomas Nelson, 1962).

several days Manson patiently observed the transformation of the structure-less *filaria* embryos into morphologically distinct larvae.

Dressed in white and dominating the center of the canvas, Manson personifies the unequal power relationship between the West and the East, temperate and tropical peoples. The placard behind Manson identifies him as port surgeon of the Customs Service. Although imposed on China by Britain and other Western powers after the Opium Wars (1839–42 and 1856–58), the Customs Service was justified in terms of the special responsibility of the West to accelerate the modernization of China through trade and cultural exchange. Depicting Manson as an "ambassador in white," the painting conveys the unmistakable impression that Manson alone as a representative of European science and medicine possesses privileged access to the workings of nature.[10] He is upright and alert to the future. By contrast, Hin-Lo is asleep. Even the stooped, un-named Chinese servant, who supports the tray of glass bottles, is oblivious to the significance of the mosquitoes.

The glass bottle that Manson inspects symbolizes the transformation of the tropical world into a far more hospitable place. By identifying the transmission of malaria, Manson helped to reveal the power of medical science to promote the development of the empire. As medical adviser to the Colonial Office, Manson used his access to the Colonial Secretary, Joseph Chamberlain, to secure the necessary financial assistance for the establishment of the London School of Tropical Medicine. The London School, which trained prospective colonial medical officers as well as private practitioners who planned to practice in the tropical world, outlived Manson. Still, the school and other national and international institutions continued Manson's legacy by mobilizing Western medical science on behalf of the tropical world. In assessing the imminent conquest of disease in the tropical world in 1962, Manson-Bahr had no doubt about who was responsible.

These [institutional milestones] in turn led to an ever-expanding development in the understanding, treatment, and prevention of the main tropical diseases — the centuries-old scourges — which has resulted in many instances in almost complete eradication, so that many countries, West Africa for example, no longer bear the unenviable reputation of being the "white man's grave," but now bid fair to develop into regular health resorts, where people can bask in the sun and wallow in the cerulean waves. The great initial impetus to this transformation and all that has led up to it is due to one man alone — Patrick Manson.[11]

Like most founding myths, the commemoration of the origins of tropical medicine in the *Mosquito Experiment with Hin-Lo* reflects a decidedly ahistorical outlook about Western medicine and science that defined the outlook of specialists in the past and continues today.[12] The image of the helpless tropical inhabitant and the resourceful European representative of medical science presumes a natural hierarchy of power and authority based on universal principles of knowledge. Of course, this presumption is both paternalistic and self-serving. But it also is misleading. It diminishes the historical role of imperialism in the making of Victorian medicine and science precisely by representing Western medicine and science in the world as the natural diffusion of universal knowledge.

The very organization of scholarly interest in the history of British medicine according to the categories of "home" and "empire" has promoted this diffusionist approach. Even valuable accounts on the social, economic, and institutional development of medicine remain surprisingly insular — so much so that it almost appears that Britain did not have an empire in the nineteenth century or that the profession was indifferent to it.[13] Only since the mid-1980s have social historians of medicine turned to the empire in earnest. At most, this new literature has revised the place of Western medical science in the empire. Recent studies of the politics of preventive medicine and public health in India,

Africa, and elsewhere have complicated, if not wholly discredited, the notion of Victorian medicine and science as an unproblematic tool of imperialism or as an unmixed blessing of colonialism.[14] Still, this very salutary examination of British medicine and science in the colonial situation has tended to reinforce, rather than dissolve, the distinction between home and empire.[15]

Manson's career in tropical medicine as a practitioner, researcher, and institution builder challenges the artificial categories of "home" and "empire." It reveals a vastly more dynamic, dialectical relationship between the imperial metropole and the periphery than has heretofore been recognized by historians of medicine. I argue that British imperialism played a central role in constituting Victorian medicine and science as a domestic institution. In a word, British medicine was imperial medicine.

My interest in tropical medicine reflects a growing body of scholarship concerned with remapping Britain as part of a wider imperial landscape. The empire was not simply out there, occupying a marginal place in the lives and imagination of British people.[16] As spectacle, it reverberated in advertisements, music-hall songs, museums, and exhibitions.[17] As a cultural and social space, it too helped to constitute fields of knowledge and social formations that had formerly been thought to be the exclusive product of a distinctive European or modern society. These range from Victorian anthropology, geology, and English literature, to modern social movements such as feminism and environmentalism, to racial differences and national identity.[18] The empire, then, was as much in Britain as it was in the periphery.

This was especially the case for British medicine. Historians have long viewed the medical register—a provision of the 1858 Medical Act—as a critical institution in legitimizing the authority and consolidating the power of regular medicine through the public identification of qualified practitioners.[19] While registration was voluntary for all practitioners until the passage of the 1886 Medical Act, this was not the case for the class of practitioners who held public positions, including those in the army, the navy, and the East India Company.[20] By tying the economic benefits of public or state employment to regular medicine, the professional establishment, ranging from the General Medical Council to medical schools and licensing bodies, undoubtedly viewed the empire as an important site for promoting the interests of the profession domestically. As it turned out, their assessment proved correct.

Over the second half of the nineteenth century, the demand for medical personnel in Britain's formal territories and its informal commercial empire was seemingly insatiable. According to one late nineteenth-century estimate, at least one-fifth of British general practitioners plied their trade in the empire in one or more capacities.[21] The Army Medical Department and the Indian and Naval Medical Services, together with the local medical services of the dependent empire, required more than two thousand practitioners or nearly 10 percent of the profession simply to attend to the needs of imperial servants and colonial subjects.[22] Other practitioners sustained Britain's global transportation and commercial system in a quasi-official capacity as medical officers on railroads, on passenger and merchant vessels, and as port surgeons. Some contracted with colonial mining concerns and plantations and/or engaged in fee-for-service practice in the burgeoning cities of white settlement in Africa, New Zealand, Australia, and Canada. Others practiced medicine in the coastal cities in Japan and China, which were forcibly opened by mid-nineteenth-century gunboat diplomacy.[23]

When Manson began his career in China in 1866 as a port surgeon in the Imperial Chinese Maritime Customs Service, he hardly expected to become the founder of tropical medicine. For him, as for many other medical graduates of Britain, overseas practice offered the only opportunity for a viable career. This was especially true at midcentury when the profession lacked a proven therapeutic technique, much less monopolized the provision of health care. In this environment, temporary and long-term employment in the empire increased the career security of individuals from the lower middle classes as well as Welsh, Scottish, and Irish doctors who lacked the social connections and capital to prosper in the "south."[24] By the end of the century, the role of the empire as an occupational safety net increased rather than diminished in importance. The dramatic expansion of Britain's territorial empire between 1880 and 1900 was paralleled by the growth in the size of the profession, which increased by 20 percent during this time. Overcrowding in the domestic medical market caused more and more practitioners to look to the empire to pursue their career ambitions.[25]

The empire also provided a critical site for defining the social position of the Victorian practitioner as well as cultural authority of British medicine. As Terence J. Johnson and Marjorie Caygill have discussed, the relatively few overseas branches of the British Medical Association (BMA) operated chiefly as advocates for the local concerns of practitioners dispersed through the empire.[26] By contrast, the medical press was far more effective in appropriating the empire as an extension of the metropolitan or domestic profession. By defending imperial doctors, who were prohibited from publicly criticizing the imperial state, the BMA's *British Medical Journal*, and its rival, the *Lancet*, both reinforced and promoted the social and economic interests of all practitioners. A steady stream of articles and special reports, as well as anonymous letters to the editor, denounced the social subordination of medical professionals to military or civilian personnel, deplored their lack of control over their time, and criticized the capricious distribution of rewards, including promotion, pay, and pension benefits.[27]

Far from being narrowly concerned with "home" matters, the medical press enhanced its authority as an organ of the profession by becoming a rhetorical medium of imperial medicine. The routine representation of the periphery as a contrasting image of medicine and health reflects the collaboration of the medical press in the cultural production of imperialism. In a range of journalistic formats, the portrayal of indigenous medicine, whether in China or in Africa, as backward made possible the representation of British medicine as effective in spite of its therapeutic inadequacies.[28] To be sure, the discourse about the "white man's grave" called into question the ability of British medicine to conquer disease. But it also offered a rationale for imperialism and colonial conquest while bolstering the cultural authority of British medicine. The image of the damaged European body or constitution, if anything, figuratively represented the limits of civilization and its absence. By representing the tropical world as diseased and atrophied, this discourse framed British society as a healthy and advanced society.[29] As Antoinette Burton has shown, British women, too, strategically used the image of the unhygienic *zenana* in India in order to promote the professionalization of female doctors at home.[30]

At the same time, the empire as a cultural and social space for the making of Victorian medicine generated as much conflict as consensus. The British empire, to be sure, was a political system of conquest and control, where power radiated from an imperial center or metropole to a subordinate periphery. Nonetheless, this framework, which accorded Europeans privileged status, did not replace the fault lines of conflict among them. This was true for a chronically underemployed medical profession, riddled with status insecurity. The very rhetorical accessibility of the empire, which played such a central role in constituting British medicine as imperial medicine, provoked heated conflicts between workers in the periphery and metropole over who was entitled to authenticate new knowledge and/or apportion scientific priority. These conflicts, which the medical press readily publicized, did not necessarily discredit imperial medical knowledge. If anything, they fostered and sustained a metropolitan audience for knowledge about the periphery.

As I show in chapters 3 and 4, the publicized conflict between investigators created a context for the reception of Manson's research into the relationship of mosquitoes to disease-causing parasites. Two and a half years before the announcement of the role of the mosquito in the life history of the *filaria* worm,

Timothy R. Lewis, a surgeon in the British Army in India, and Thomas S. Cobbold, a London-based natural scientist, engaged in an intense dispute over the priority of discovery of the immature and adult stages of the worm. Rather than immediately seeking publicity for his discovery, Manson solicited the approval of Cobbold and Lewis. Cobbold endorsed the experimental basis of the role of the mosquito as intermediary host, while Lewis expressed his doubts. Their contradictory assessments in the press not only marked an extension of their public feud but also made Manson's discovery newsworthy.

Later, Manson harnessed the medical press to promote his mosquito-malaria theory after returning to Britain permanently in 1889 after nearly twenty years in China. Even though Manson never left Britain to investigate or demonstrate his theory, he created a context for the discovery of the transmission of the malaria parasite through metropolitan publicity. By publicizing the ongoing, though inconclusive, investigations of Ronald Ross in India in professional venues that received press coverage, Manson literally made the theory interesting to the metropolitan profession. While Manson's practice of promoting Ross's incomplete research generated criticism, he nonetheless succeeded in mobilizing official and professional support for the theory by portraying the mosquito-malaria relationship as British science. In the context of increasing competition from continental rivals in the world, this appeal to patriotism elevated the demonstration of his theory to a matter of national honor. These efforts, which led to a special malaria research appointment for Ross in India, culminated in the discovery of the transmission of malaria by the bite of the mosquito.

This milestone in British medical science took place against the backdrop of a major crisis in the profession. By the 1890s, the size of the profession had ballooned by 20 percent since 1880. Just as earlier in the century, overcrowding simply encouraged more practitioners to seek occupational safe havens, especially in the colonial medical services of the dependent empire. The low opportunity costs of colonial appointments made them comparatively attractive to underemployed practitioners. The Colonial Office, which recruited general practitioners for the empire, expected at least one approved or registerable qualification and permitted imperial doctors to serve as long as they liked. Commissions in the Army Medical Department and the Indian and Naval Medical Services were more demanding. They required selection based on competitive examination, followed by six months of mandatory instruction at Netley for the Army and India Service or Haslar for the Naval Medical Department and a legally binding multiple-year commitment.

These liberal conditions seemingly served the mutual needs of general practitioners and the imperial state. They broadened the pool of potential applicants for colonial service while making appointments in the empire relatively easy to secure. In fact, these conditions barely disguised an uneven power relationship between the Colonial Office and the profession. The availability of qualified practitioners enabled the Colonial Office to satisfy the personnel needs of a geographically diverse and decentralized territorial empire cheaply and with only a tenuous commitment to practitioners. Colonial governments, in turn, maximized the labor of imperial doctors as primary-care givers chiefly through the exercise of wide discretionary authority, performance-based financial incentives, and the strict regulation of the privilege of private practice.

Before the 1890s, the profession through the medical press decried these conditions as incommensurate with the education and training of medical professionals. Predictably, proposals surfaced in the press for professionalizing the colonial medical services when overcrowding in the late nineteenth century enhanced the leverage of the Colonial Office. Those practitioners who argued for professionalization sought to assert the power of the metropolitan profession over the empire through the creation of a specialized body of knowledge, certified by medical schools and mediated by qualified practitioners. By organizing entry and career emoluments around tropical medicine, the profession in turn hoped to raise the social position of imperial doctors as salaried employees. In spite of the demand for reform, the profession still lacked the power to realize it.

The metropolitan discourse on tropical medicine interested Colonial Secretary Joseph Chamberlain, a leading proponent for the late nineteenth-century policy of *constructive imperialism*. This policy called for the active leadership of the imperial state in the economic development of Britain's empire, especially the dependent tropical empire long known as the "white man's grave." But imperial officials preferred to approach the problem of disease in the dependent empire by improving the efficiency of imperial doctors as primary-care givers rather than enhancing their social power. As medical adviser to the Colonial Office, Manson provided the means to achieve this end by proposing the Royal Albert Docks Branch Hospital of the Seamen's Hospital Society as a special school for prospective imperial doctors. By designating the London School of Tropical Medicine as the single portal of entry into the colonial medical services, the Colonial Office asserted its power as a major recruiter and employer of practitioners in the metropole. This was small comfort to medical schools and other interested professional groups, which vainly attempted to reverse the decision.

This uneven power relationship between the imperial state and the metropolitan profession had long-term consequences for British medical science. By maximizing the labor of imperial doctors as primary-care givers, colonial governments were able to service European personnel and their families and, as resources permitted, colonial subjects. This use of medical personnel, however, created the conditions for the domestication of the study of disease in the empire in Britain itself. Established in 1903 at the prompting of Chamberlain, the Tropical Diseases Research Fund enabled contributing colonies to complement their emphasis on primary care. It, too, generated an important new source of funding for metropolitan medical science. This net transfer of resources from the empire institutionalized research science at the London School of Tropical Medicine and elsewhere in Britain while laying the foundation for the hegemonic authority of metropolitan specialist science over disease in the tropical world.

1

The Making of an Imperial Doctor

*Also please do not change "England" to "Scotland": the sense of the pas-
sage is that he left home too young to have made acquaintance with any
big men at headquarters (which is London, not Scotland) who might have
been a weight onto his feet afterwards and might have done for him what
he [Manson] did for Ross. So it should be "England." Scotland would be
grotesque, since all Soctchmen come to England for their opportunity.*

COLONEL A. ALCOCK TO P. H. MANSON-BAHR
8 October 1926, regarding their biography of Patrick Manson

*Quinine is as valuable to a man shivering with ague as a piece of grey
shirting; and when he knows this he will ask for it, and get it. But if
grey shirtings were only to be got from one or two charitable individuals, either the mass would probably remain ignorant of their existence,
or the charity of these individuals be soon exhausted. Private enterprise
would be choked by the give-away-for-nothing system of the philanthro-
pist, and certainly clothes for the millions would not be forthcoming. Left
to the wholesome influence of supply and demand, we know how mar-
velous has been the result, and so it should be with quinine.*

PATRICK MANSON
Medical and Surgical Report for the Amoy (China) Missionary Hospital for 1873

AT first sight, the village of Takow on the island of Taiwan (or Formosa, as it was then known) appears to be an unlikely place for Patrick Manson to have launched his career in medicine. Takow could not have been farther from his birthplace in Oldmeldrum, Aberdeenshire, or from his medical training at Aberdeen University in Scotland. But Manson's career path was hardly an anomaly. It goes without saying that most graduates of English, Irish, and Scottish medical schools would have preferred to pursue lucrative careers as London consultants. Many tried, but few succeeded. This sobering reality did little to check demand for medical training after 1850. Most toiled away as providers in a competitive domestic medical market. Yet, as Britain's formal territorial and informal commercial empire grew, an increasing number of practitioners pursued their careers abroad. Many sought the security of a salaried appointment in the state services, that is, the Army Medical Department, the Indian Medical Service, the Naval Medical Service, or the colonial medical services of the dependent empire. Others served on merchant and passenger vessels in hopes of a better situation. Still others preferred to gamble on the promise of cultivating markets for medicine in British colonies or in Britain's spheres of influence. Regardless of their occupational status, as a group they practiced medicine as imperial physicians and, consequently, participated in the transformation of Victorian medicine into imperial medicine. As this chapter will show, Manson was both a product and an agent of this process.

The Making of a Doctor in Victorian Scotland

In a parish church in the farm town of Old Machar in northeast Scotland, Patrick Blaikie, a retired Royal Navy surgeon, gave his eighteen-year-old daughter Elizabeth away in marriage on 16 June 1842.[1] The groom was John Manson, a thirty-five-year-old property owner and bank agent for the North of Scotland Banking Company in Oldmeldrum, a prosperous farm town in the county of Aberdeenshire.[2] Shortly after their marriage, John and Elizabeth moved to a large four-bedroom house with surrounding farmland on Cromlet Hill in Oldmeldrum. The Manson family quickly outgrew their home. First came John Blaikie in June 1843. Patrick followed him in October 1844. Forbes was born in March 1846, David in July 1847, Margaret Knight in November 1848, Alexander Livingstone in July 1850, Elisabeth Livingstone in August 1852, Helen in May 1854, and Alice in January 1856.[3]

In 1859, John and Elizabeth relocated the family to 22 King Street in the eastern portion of Aberdeen. Their decision to migrate to the city, some twenty miles from Oldmeldrum, conformed to a well-established pattern of internal migration in northeastern Scotland. As the regional center of banking, higher education, insurance, and law, Aberdeen was the magnet for the growing population in the hinterland of the county. Between 1801 and 1851, Aberdeen's population nearly tripled, from 26,900 to 72,000.[4]

In moving, John and Elizabeth gave up the rural gentility of Cromlet Hill for a plain townhouse in a middle-class district of the city. The loss in charm was more than made up for in space. The twelve rooms comfortably accommodated a household consisting of two adults and eight growing children. Three female servants lightened the work for Elizabeth. If the number of servants is taken as an index of social class, King Street included a wide spectrum of the middle class. Next-door to the Mansons lived a grocer and his wife, who employed one servant. At 36 King Street, George Morrison, a doctor, and his wife shared their one servant with a traveling-salesman lodger. Farther down the block, customs collector Daniel Briston and his wife and two sons looked after themselves.[5]

Like other families of the burgeoning Aberdeen middle class, John and Elizabeth regarded a university education as the best means of securing their sons' social advancement. (The eldest son, John, apparently died young, as virtually nothing is known about him.) This concern accounts for their decision to enroll Patrick, David, and Forbes in West End Academy, New Town Grammar School, and the Gymnasium, respectively.[6] Unlike locally supported burgh schools, which concentrated on commercial subjects, these proprietary schools were geared to prepare their students for the entrance examination of the recently reconstituted University of Aberdeen.[7]

In preparing Patrick for this examination, John and Elizabeth had already determined what career he was to pursue. A medical degree offered the best value for achieving financial independence and social advancement. Although Scotland's universities as well as its medical corporations produced far more doctors than could be assimilated in the small medical market, many found employment by migrating south to England. The reciprocity provision of the 1858 Medical Act, which placed Scottish medical degrees and qualifications on the same footing as those from England, probably made migration all the more attractive.[8] For those graduates without prospects in either Scotland or England, there was always the vast British empire. The demand for medical personnel continued, whether in the various state and colonial medical services or for private practitioners in the growing colonies of white settlement in Australia, New Zealand, Canada, and South Africa.

Manson's success as a medical student at Aberdeen University showed the wisdom of his parents' decision. After passing the preliminary examination in 1861, he attended lectures and demonstrations on anatomy, botany, chemistry, clinical medicine and surgery, *materia medica*, medical jurisprudence, and midwifery. Between April and July 1862, Manson obtained his pharmacological experience; he completed his surgical and medical apprenticeship at the Royal Infirmary at Aberdeen and Edinburgh the following spring and summer.[9] His two professional examinations, in 1863 and 1864, were each recognized as "deserving of commendation."[10] In 1865, he received his baccalaureate degree in medicine with honorable distinction. He then collected material for his master's thesis while working as an assistant medical officer at a lunatic asylum in Durham County at Winterton.[11] After he submitted his thesis, entitled "On a Peculiar Affection of the Internal Carotid Artery in Connection with Diseases of the Brain," the university conferred Manson's medical degree in 1866.[12]

Excellence at medical school did not translate into career success either in Aberdeen or in England. It is likely that even before Manson received his medical degree, he had decided that a career in Britain was beyond his reach. Manson passed his third medical examination three months shy of his twentieth birthday; twenty was the minimum age for practicing legally (Figure 2). During this period, he visited his uncle in London, where he read and visited hospitals and museums.[13] To be sure, being at the center of the medical profession in England was an exciting experience for a young man living away from parents and siblings for the first time. But it was also a sobering look at his future career.

Launching a career in London was not easy, nor was success guaranteed. As Jeanne Peterson and Anne Digby have shown, the fee-for-service medical market was highly competitive. The bulk of the population relied either on home remedies or on those purchased over the counter at the chemist's. Private practitioners faced competition from new institutions, such as voluntary hospitals and cash-dispensaries, which emerged in the nineteenth century to deliver health care to the laboring and lower middle classes. While these hospitals played a vital role as sites for medical and surgical training and innovation, they shrank the size of the fee-paying market. Unlike voluntary hospitals, cash-dispensaries democratized health care by offering low-cost medicine at a fixed charge. But retailing medicine, based on economies of scale, diminished the ability of other practitioners to maximize the value of their services. For the comparatively few practitioners who serviced a middle- and upper-class clientele, competition was equally intense. While social connections and economic resources enabled them to buy into and cultivate a practice, the sheer abundance of doctors made retaining and recruiting new clients an ongoing and uncertain process.[14]

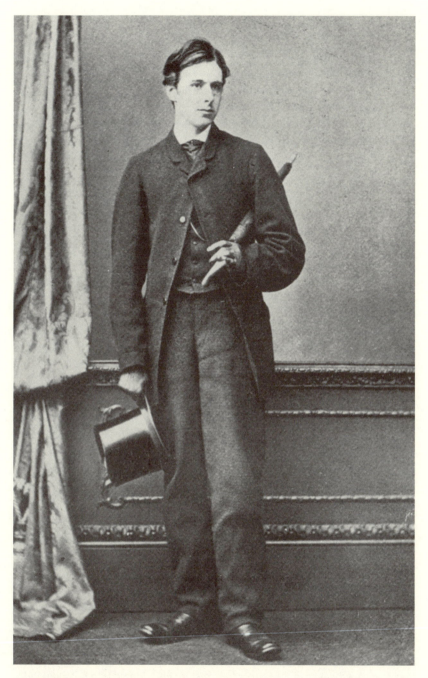

2. Patrick Manson in 1864. From Philip H. Manson-Bahr and A. Alcock, *The Life and Work of Sir Patrick Manson* (London: Cassell, 1927).

Besides a highly competitive medical market, Manson faced another obstacle, namely, metropolitan discrimination against Scottish professional qualifications. In spite of the reciprocity provision of the Medical Act of 1858, candidates for the leading London hospitals and public posts were expected to possess a qualification from the Royal College of Surgeons or the Royal College of Physicians.[15] This expectation had little to do with the quality of training in Scotland; rather, it reflected the institutional power of the Royal Colleges. By the second half of the century, College men dominated the senior hospital ranks and, in turn, made membership in the Colleges virtually obligatory for those seeking hospital positions and public posts.[16] For graduates of Scottish medical schools, the power of the Colleges not only unfairly questioned the integrity of their medical training but also increased the costs of pursuing a career in London.[17] Some looked for less prestigious posts either in the metropole or in the provinces. Still others saw their opportunities outside of Britain altogether. In 1866, Manson secured an appointment as a port surgeon in the Imperial Maritime Customs Service.

The Imperial Chinese Maritime Customs Service was not a part of the formal British empire per se. As the name implies, the service, which collected duties and maintained the shipping facilities in designated ports, fell under the authority of the emperor of China. In truth, the customs service gave expression to the ascendancy of Britain and the Western powers after China's defeat in the Opium Wars (1838–42 and 1856–58). These wars grew out of China's attempt to curb the importation of illicit Indian-grown opium. Britain used its leverage after these wars not to rule China as a colony but to secure the Chinese imperial state's sanction for a wider field of Western trade in designated ports by treaty (see map).[18] As a product of gunboat diplomacy, the customs service supplanted a highly regulated indigenous system of trade whereby Western merchants had been confined to Canton and dependent on native intermediaries. Led by Inspector-General Robert Hart, an Anglo-Irishman, the service facilitated East-West trade and served as an influential conduit of Western science and technology in China well into the twentieth century.

When looking back on the start of his career, Manson recalled that he had sought an appointment as a port surgeon in the Imperial Chinese Maritime Customs Service because of his "adventurous spirit."[19] It is more likely that when Manson surveyed his career prospects, occupational emigration appeared to be a risk worth taking. He did not seek a metropolitan corporate qualification. For a medical graduate eager to translate his training into financial independence, a customs appointment possessed several advantages. Unlike those seeking entry into the Army Medical Department, the Indian Medical Service, and the Naval Medical Service, whose requirements included passing a com-

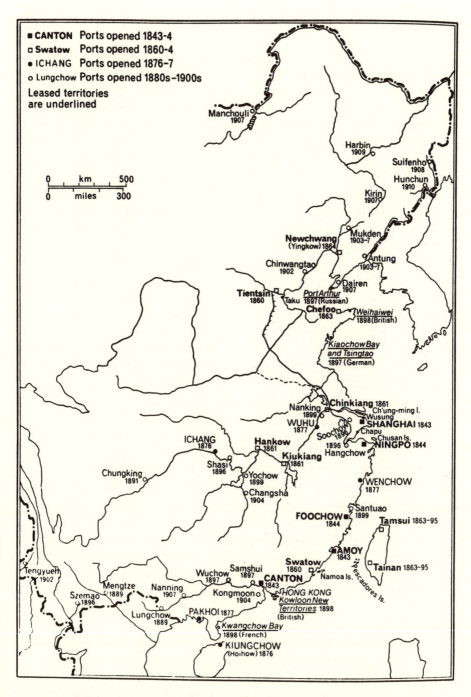

Growth of treaty ports. From Denis Twitchett and John K. Fairbank, *The Cambridge History of China*, vol. 10, *Late Ch'ing, 1800–1911*, pt. 1, p. 512.

petitive examination and completing a mandatory course of instruction, port surgeons were expected to have only medical and surgical qualifications.

The financial prospects were also encouraging. As the unofficial medical personnel of the treaty ports, customs officers mainly certified the health of arriving merchant seamen and departing emigrants. The fees, which were paid by shipowners and emigrants, could be considerable at busy ports. Beyond these fees, China offered unique conditions for an enterprising practitioner to build a prosperous private practice. Apart from missionary doctors, port surgeons had the advantage of being among the only Western doctors in treaty ports. The health-care needs of the foreign settlement communities as well as the merchant seamen provided a ready, if not captive, clientele. Finally, as liminal spaces between the East and the West, treaty ports offered a potentially vast market for Western medicine in the local Chinese population.[20]

Manson's decision to seek his fortunes outside of Britain was not unusual for an Aberdeen graduate. Ten out of nineteen honors graduates in medicine from Aberdeen University pursued imperial service. Four entered the Army Medical Department, one obtained a commission in the Naval Medical Service, and five joined the Indian Medical Service. Between 1860 and 1900, at least 18 percent of Scottish-born Aberdeen medical graduates ventured abroad. Well over half emigrated to colonies of white settlement in either South Africa or Australia. Another 12 percent obtained commissions in the state services or the colonial services of the dependent empire.[21]

After a three-month voyage that took Manson from Southampton to Gibraltar, Malta, Alexandria, Point de Galle, Penang, Singapore, and Hong Kong, he was unceremoniously dropped at the beach of Takow on the southwest side of the island of Formosa.[22] For Manson, there was no turning back. As the first family member to obtain a university education and pursue a professional calling, he would have found it, at the very least, a humbling experience to return to Scotland with little evidence of success. Rather than abetting his "adventurous spirit," it is likely that this stark reality engendered in Manson an eye for opportunities and the will for realizing them. As his subsequent China career will show, for Manson, medicine was not so much a calling as a business.

Transforming Victorian Medicine into Imperial Medicine:
Manson and the Business of Western Medicine in South China

For four years, Manson toiled in Takow before moving across the straits of Formosa to the island of Amoy in 1871. Opened to foreign trade in 1865, Takow was not an ideal trade center. It lacked a wide bay, and the inner harbor was shallow. Nor was reaching the inner harbor easy. Ocean vessels had to negotiate a strip of channel, bounded on each side by rocky surfaces, that narrowed to sixty yards across. In addition to being relatively inaccessible, the port exported little besides sugar, turmeric, and sesame seeds. The prohibition on the export of rice deprived it of the ability to sell a commodity in high demand on the mainland and in part accounts for the small extent of its imports.[23]

Like the port of Takow, financial opportunities for Manson were not particularly encouraging. Health examination fees were few and far between. During an eight-month period in 1866–67, for example, Manson examined 130 crewmembers on eleven vessels.[24] During some months of the year, the port was largely inactive. Nor were the prospects for private practice any better. The foreign population numbered thirty-eight, according to one estimate for 1882, and it is doubtful that there was much of a market for fee-based Western medicine to be found in the impoverished rural countryside.[25] With plenty of time on his hands, Manson developed into a sportsman, shooting snipe, fishing, riding, and exploring the interior of the island.

From Manson's vantage point, opportunity lay across the Formosa straits on the island of Amoy. Located at the mouth of the Min River in the Bay of Hiu Tau, Amoy was a bustling port for the inland city of Ch'angchow and a dynamic regional center for South China trade. Manson could not overlook the Chinese junks and lorches in the straits, forming a veritable floating bridge where agricultural produce and manufactured goods were exchanged between the mainland and the numerous smaller islands that dotted the bay. Moreover, Amoy's deep port made it an important transit point for European vessels. Some six European steam-vessel companies regularly plied the coastal waters from the straits of Formosa to Hong Kong, Swatow, and Foochow. Amoy's trade activity dwarfed that of Takow. In 1864, some 661 vessels cleared at Amoy, registering 210,539 tons. The following year, the number of vessels increased by 101, bringing the tonnage to 278,319.[26]

Besides being an important entrepôt for trade, Amoy (along with Swatow) was a major point of departure for emigrants from Fukien.[27] Rising population pressure, as well as soaring inflation and political unrest, pushed waves of Fukien residents from the hinterland to the coast. These "push factors" coincided with an external "pull factor": the pressing need for cheap labor in the Pacific basin and undeveloped regions of the Americas after the abolition of the African slave trade.[28] This movement of people proved to be particularly lucrative for a customs officer: All emigrants destined for the Spanish Philippines, the Dutch Indies, French Indochina, and the British Straits Settlements (modern-day Malaysia) were required to possess a vaccination certificate.[29] In 1871, Manson moved to Amoy.

After Takow, Amoy was a veritable gold mine for fees. Manson examined and treated nearly 740 sailors in 1872–73 alone.[30] Considering Amoy's location as a transit point for emigration to the Pacific basin, he undoubtedly did a brisk business in health examinations as well.[31] These later fees were only part of Manson's income. In a short time, Manson succeeded in cultivating a large private practice. By trading on his position as a port surgeon, he contracted out his services to shipowners. As a resident of the neighboring island of Kulangsu, where most of the one hundred or more Westerners lived, Manson included the British consul among his clients.[32] Perhaps the most lucrative source of Manson's income was his cash-dispensary in Amoy, which catered mainly to the local Chinese population.

The success of Manson's dispensary not only underscores his enterprise but also reveals the latent tension between two Western imperial enterprises in China: medicine and religion. Manson's for-profit dispensary originated in his position as surgeon and physician in charge of the local nonprofit mission hospital of the Presbyterian Church of England. The mission hospital symbolized the growing presence of Protestant missionary activity in China after the Opium Wars and the importance of Western medicine in the promotion of Christianity. Chinese suspicion had long frustrated the Pauline mission to convert souls. Unlike Chinese doctors, whose customs forbade invasive procedures, Western doctors had the benefit of centuries of anatomical knowledge about and surgical experience with the body. The mission hospital provided an ideal opportunity to dissipate suspicion through effective surgical intervention while preaching the virtues of Christian religion.

Daniel MacGowan, an American medical missionary of the Presbyterian Church in 1842, pointed out to students at the College of Surgeons of New York the advantages of a medical missionary over a "minister of the gospel." "The physician has access to communities and families in heathen lands as a missionary laborer, where the evangelist is not permitted to enter. He has it in his power at once, to give to the distrustful heathen [a] palpable demonstration of the benevolence of his errand. This he can do with comparatively an imperfect knowledge of the sufferer's language." The task was far more daunting for a missionary without medical training. "The minister of the gospel, on the other hand, can do nothing of his appropriate work without language. He is compelled to toil long, and amidst obloquy and reproach, before he can convince his hearers that he is actuated by disinterested motives, the existence of which class of feelings it is exceedingly difficult for the pagan to believe."[33]

Still, the missionary enterprise in Amoy faced a chronic shortage of practitioners. James C. Hepburn, who was sponsored by the American Board of Commissioners of Foreign Mission, lasted only two years (1843–45). The tenure of William Henry Cumming (1842–47) was only one year longer. Nor could the mission hospital, which was supported by the Amoy merchant community, retain its missionaries. Dr. James Young returned to Britain in 1854 after three years of service. Young's successor, Dr. John Carnegie, arrived in 1859 but died in 1862.[34]

Manson's appointment as surgeon and physician in charge of the mission hospital in 1871 was a marriage of convenience. After years of disruptions in hospital personnel, Manson afforded a measure of stability: He was not going anywhere. He honed his skills as a surgeon and doctor at the mission hospital. As the principal site for the Chinese encounter with Western medicine, the mission hospital provided Manson with an ideal vantage point from which to assess the viability of a market for his services. This latter interest ensured that Manson's association with the mission hospital would be a source of tension with its European personnel.

At issue was a much wider conflict between religion and medicine over the function of medicine in China. Even within the missionary movement itself, the union of medicine and the ministry proved to be a contentious one. Some viewed the demands of delivering medicine as incompatible with a narrow conception of mission work. It was for this reason that William Lockhart, who served as a nonministerial medical missionary for the London Missionary Society in China, stressed that medical missionaries should be laymen.[35] Still others recommended a middle way of sorts by subordinating healing to the conversion of souls. "The medical missionary should have great singleness of purpose," Daniel MacGowan insisted, "never allowing his secondary object, the healing of disease, and the promotion of science, to become his primary one; this honor should in his mind belong only to the conversion of souls, else in the end he will prove a stumbling block to the heathen, and a scandal to the Church. He must literally give himself and that for life; he must resolve to live poor, and to die poor, looking for his reward to the great Physician of our souls, and be content for the present, with the rich luxury of doing good." [36]

The metropolitan profession was ambivalent about the role of medicine in the missionary project in China. On the one hand, the portrayal of Chinese medicine as spurious helped to constitute the identity of British medicine as legitimate in relation to alternative medical regimes in Europe. "We are so often stupefied with the pretensions and amazed at the absurd theories of English and continental quacks," a reviewer of a travel narrative about China opined,

"that it is a refreshing amusement to go further afield and note the unsophisti-
cated follies of a race of men who really believe the nonsense which they talk,
and who are accredited with a curative power which is held by millions to be
not inferior to that of the homoeopath or kinesipath [*sic*]." [37]

Similarly, to the extent that the missionary discourse portrayed Chinese
medicine as backward, it reinforced the image of China as an atrophied civilization while helping to construct British medicine as a symbol of the West, that is,
as modern and progressive. "Apart from the moral interest attaching to medical missionaries," a *Lancet* review of medical missionary reports from China
and India noted, "it is impossible to look upon the labours of medical missionaries, and upon their contention with old forms of medicine and civilization,
with anything but much pleasure. We venture to believe that when the history of
the first effective impression made by Western nations upon the old and effete
notions of the East comes to be written, a most honourable, if not the very first,
page will be reserved for an account of the labours of the first men who went
out in the capacity of medical missionaries." [38]

On the other hand, charitable medicine in China posed a serious threat to
the economic interests of all practitioners. Before the Edinburgh Medical Missionary Society, William Swan acknowledged the value of charitable medicine.
However, in the same breath, he discouraged competition between the medical missionary and the private practitioner. "We would deem it inexpedient to
send a Medical Missionary to any of the great cities of the East where European and American physicians or surgeons are stationed in sufficient number
to meet the demand made upon them by the natives around. . . . It would evidently be improper to send a Medical Missionary (whose services among the
native population must be in general gratuitous) where a private practitioner
has established himself, and must live by his profession." [39]

After the financial disappointment at Takow, Manson had little patience
with the evangelical purpose of mission medicine. In his reports, directed at
the largely merchant benefactors of the hospital, he explicitly dissociated the
practice of Western medicine from the missionary enterprise. During his first
year in charge of the hospital, a poison-pill scare caused the usual number of
applicants to decline. But Manson reported how effective surgical treatment
for a range of conditions, including the first known excision of a tumor from
the scrotum, had restored local confidence in the hospital as an institution of
"disinterested benevolence." "Great numbers knew of this and we were most
anxious for its success. Should one patient [have] died after this operation, this
combined with the disturbing effects of these rumors would have almost been
fatal to the reputation of the Hospital." [40]

The results of mission medicine were decidedly mixed, however. The growth in applicants seeking treatment for scrotal disease after 1871 demonstrated the promise of Western medicine in China, as Manson reported: "Till August 1871 no case of the sort had been operated on in Amoy since the foundation of the Hospital, then by accident a man was brought to submit and his case terminating successfully, others were led to apply for removal of the same disease; so that last year [1873] no fewer than 18 cases were operated on, making altogether 31 cases in the short space of two years and a half." Yet there was little or no evidence that the Chinese appreciated the superiority of Western medical treatment. "Something theatrical as the removal of the stone from a bladder, the excision of a tumor and such like proceedings," Manson volunteered, "impress the ignorant more than something infinitely more difficult and wonderful, such as the elaborate diagnosis of some internal disease, which a modern physician, the inheritor of centuries of patient investigation and scientific intention, can make." If anything, this indifference to the Western healing art reinforced a preference for Chinese medicine. "Most people recover from most sicknesses whether by European or Chinese physicians. The Chinaman can point thus to numerous so called cures by his own medicines, and declines to abandon the old, so long as there is what he considers known good to it, for the new with unknown and indefinite evil in it." [41]

Manson did not attribute the preference for indigenous medicine to Chinese pride or prejudice but rather to what he deemed to be the pernicious effects of charitable medicine. Unlike Chinese medicine, Western medical treatment had no value assigned to it. Even if it was superior, there was no basis for comparison because one came with a price and the other did not. Manson complained that mission medicine was used by the poor but was not valued by the rich. "The poor who cannot pay . . . are in a measure forced to apply to us. Coolies, opium smokers, soldiers, peddlers, farm labourers, prostitutes, sailors, beggars, waifs and strays they think, whatever they may say, that any doctor is better than none." Others sought out assistance from the mission hospital not based on the authority of the Western physician but as a last resort. "People in the last stages of an incurable disease apply to us thinking [that although] their own doctors have failed to cure them there may be a chance with the foreigner." [42]

There was a self-serving, if not hypocritical, quality to Manson's jeremiad against mission medicine. Medical missions allowed him to hone his skills as a surgeon, and they exposed the Chinese population to Western medicine. In truth, Manson deployed this distorted representation of mission medicine to justify his decision to open a consulting room and a cash-dispensary a year after joining the hospital. This initiative, he explained in his 1873 report, was designed "to bring our art into more favourable consideration amongst the higher class of Chinese." By adopting Chinese practices in attending and billing patients, Manson boasted, "I have had mandarins, shopkeepers, and even members of the native faculty amongst my patients."[43] Success made Manson even less tolerant of charitable medicine.

Absurd systems like gratuitous dispensing of advice and medicines to any one who likes to apply, or the forcing of it on them should be abandoned. Our art of science should be presented as something worth a price, and in the same way as their Doctors come to them and to us—if this is done I have no doubt we will get a still firmer hold. It is said that the Emperor of China did not appreciate the handsome present of a railway made to him the other day; had he bought it he probably would.[44]

Throughout his early association with the mission hospital, Manson possessed the tacit approval of the merchant benefactors of the hospital. Otherwise, it is unlikely that he would have maintained his association with the hospital while operating his cash-dispensary. Even though merchant communities played an important role in subsidizing mission hospitals and other related missionary activities, it would be misleading to infer that they wholly embraced the missionary enterprise. The evangelical work of missionaries was one area that destabilized the delicate relationship between local Chinese and the foreign community. Proselytizing provoked a generalized hostility toward foreigners; also, the religious toleration clause of the Treaty of Tientsin enabled Chinese converts to circumvent the mainstays of China's local social and political authorities, the gentry and bureaucracy.[45] Further, growing missionary opposition to the opium trade jeopardized a valuable source of revenue for American and British merchants.[46] These factors may well have led to changing the name from Amoy Missionary Hospital to Amoy Chinese Hospital in 1873.

This new name reflected more substantive changes taking place inside and outside the mission hospital. As surgeon and doctor in charge, Manson took it upon himself to promote the free-enterprise ethic among the hospital trainees, who were expected to carry the Christian gospel back to their villages. In subverting the aim of missionary medicine, Manson freely admitted that several students, whom he had outfitted, had left the service of the hospital to pursue a more financially rewarding practice of medicine.[47] "I tapped a branch of society hitherto incredulous and estranged. Chintong who used to be in charge of the Chinese Hospital acts as apothecary and treats the simpler cases, and I believe the prospect of more remunerative employment there will have a stimulating effect on the boys and young men employed at the Native Hospital."[48]

Of course, not everyone approved of Manson's activities. In a letter to the *Chinese Recorder*, the Reverend William M'Gregor tartly reported that the hospital had ceased being "an agency [for] the spread of the Gospel." Chinese hospital assistants viewed medicine as means to make money, not to save souls. "We heard many stories of patients finding it for their interest to fee the assistants, and were on more than one occasion told that the treatment they sometimes met with was calculated to do anything but recommend Christianity to them." On preaching days, Chinese missionaries were reminded that they "had no control of the hospital, that it was maintained by the mercantile community, and that when they came to preach they were there only on sufferance." M'Gregor predictably severed the mission's connection with the "management of the new non-Christian institution." [49]

* * *

The integrity of Britain's empire and imperial interests was based on individual choices. As Manson's early career shows, these choices generated powerful ties that linked the metropole and the periphery. Like other doctors in Britain who lacked career prospects, Manson sought greener pastures abroad as a port surgeon for the Imperial Chinese Maritime Customs Service. As a medical practitioner in China, Manson served an institution that symbolized Western hegemony and facilitated the penetration of Western commercial relationships. Leveraging his association with the local mission hospital, Manson cultivated a new market for Western medicine by opening a cash-dispensary in Amoy. Financial success only deepened Manson's involvement in the British imperial project.

Before taking his first furlough to Britain in 1874, Manson assisted the career of his brother David, who had just graduated from Aberdeen University in 1872. David substituted for Manson during his absence before beginning his own short-lived career as a customs port surgeon at Takow in 1875. With David managing his practice, Manson could lead the life of a man of independent means in Britain.

2
Transforming Colonial Knowledge into Imperial Knowledge

The Isolation of the Mosquito as Intermediary
Host of the *Filaria* Worm

RETURNING to Britain, Manson participated in the dense circulation of people between the imperial periphery and the metropole. Furloughs, or leaves of absence, represented an important social institution that sustained Britain's imperial culture at home and in its wider empire. Official and semi-official positions, as well as those associated with trading companies and plantations, usually provided for approved leaves of absence after the completion of a fixed number of years of service.[1] During this period, imperial servants could receive from two months to two years of leave while drawing full or partial salary. Both as a reward for service and as a promise of job security, the furlough made British as well as European imperialism a practical possibility: It encouraged the growth of a relatively stable imperial workforce.

The furlough also facilitated the domestication of the empire. After a protracted absence, imperial servants returned as visitors to their native land. Still, the homecoming of sons, fathers, nephews, and uncles underscored the emotional and personal ties that linked home and community to the wider imperial project. These ties grew through marriage between imperial servants and British women. Indeed, Manson's own marriage during his furlough was no exception. If anything, such unions reveal the complementary demographic realities that made them desirable, namely, the scarcity of European women in the empire and their surplus at home.

The yearlong furlough provided Manson with an occasion not only to deepen his personal stake in the empire but also to recast his understanding of the cause of elephantiasis, a disease endemic to South China. At first sight, the library of the British Museum seems an unlikely place for Manson to learn about the existence of *Filaria sanguinis hominis*. Yet, in all but name, the British Museum was an imperial institution. Its vast and growing collection of books and periodicals made the library a repository for the cultural production of knowledge about the empire. This was especially important for imperial doctors who, dispersed throughout the empire, lacked regular access to a medical library. By providing imperial doctors, such as Manson, with a space to compare their own colonial medical knowledge with what was known elsewhere in the empire, the library functioned not only as a reference source but also as a space for the production of imperial knowledge itself. Manson's later isolation of the mosquito as the intermediary host of *F. sanguinis hominis* in China in 1877 continued a process that had begun in Bloomsbury.

Finding Love in London

For unattached European males, treaty ports in China offered few opportunities for lasting romance—at least with single European women. Given the military and commercial nature of Europe's relationship with China in the nineteenth century, the scarcity of single European women is not surprising. Imperial service was mainly men's work. The British army, navy, and merchant marine consisted of single males who were recruited disproportionately from the working classes. Their contact with China was instrumental, transient, and strictly regulated. To the extent that Western women were present, they usually accompanied imperial professionals—ranging from military officials to diplomatic and senior customs personnel to merchants and missionaries—as wives and daughters (in other words, as dependents).

As Anne Stoler and others have argued, the regulation of the presence of European women was no accident.[2] This practice enabled imperial and corporate officials to control the social contours of the Western presence in China while reinforcing hierarchies of power within the foreign settlement community. This was the case for men such as Manson, who occupied the ambiguous social space between transient and semipermanent imperial personnel. They were older than university students but not yet middle-aged. Their association with important institutions such as the Imperial Chinese Maritime Customs Service made them members of the foreign community. Undoubtedly, the preference for middle-class bachelors reflected a desire among customs officials to ensure a high standard of living and, by extension, buttress white prestige in China. However, there was a cost associated with the seven-year marriage prohibition in the customs service, namely, marginality within the foreign settlement community.[3] Bachelors lived apart from their superiors, and strict social conventions mediated their contact with married European women.

Paul King, sometime customs commissioner in China, recalled the social distinctions that existed in the foreign settlement community of Swatow, a small coastal port south of Amoy.

Swatow suffered then, as it does now, from divided interests. The foreign settlement is on each side of the harbour and separated by a mile or so of not always easily navigated tidal water. Consequently, social barriers had grown up. It was more "tony" to live on one side than on the other. We of the Customs were also divided. Our Chief, the Commissioner, lived on the "tony" side, while his four assistants dwelt over the Custom House amidst Chinese and business conditions. Another social disability for dwellers on the Swatow side lay in the fact that the married people—mostly seniors—all dwelt on the opposite side at Kahchio.[4]

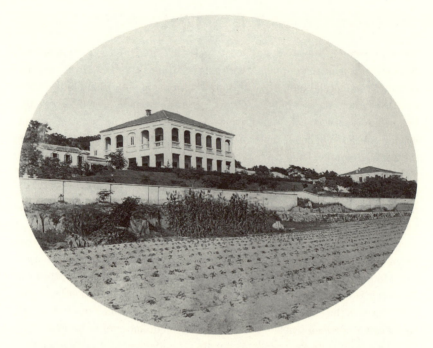

3. The clubhouse, Amoy, China. From Wellcome Institute Library, London.

The situation was little better in Amoy. Kulangsu served as the unofficial home of the foreign community. Members of the consular staff, leading merchants, and the missionary community not only made the island their home but also organized their social life around the clubhouse (Figure 3). There was not much for single men to do. One treaty port guidebook noted, "Socially, it is not liked as a residence on account of its limited foreign community and the small number of ladies who have found their way thither." [5]

This social segregation among foreigners in treaty ports created a distinctive bachelor culture. King described this culture in Swatow as the "Jambarree spirit." "Every now and then we were invited over to rather solemn dinner parties followed by whist, but as a rule most Swatowites had to shift for themselves in matters of social intercourse on a bachelor basis, with the inevitable result that the 'Jambarree' spirit was ever present. Sometimes wearisomely so, card-playing—chiefly poker—was also much in vogue, while the night side of Chinese life was to be had for the asking all around us. It was a strange enough environment for white youth fresh from home." [6]

The sexual lives of Western men in China reflected the social hierarchy within the foreign community. Many, particularly among army and navy personnel, turned to brothels. Better-situated men in the customs service, as well as traders, formed long-term relationships with *mui-tsai*, a special class of Chinese women who provided sex, companionship, or domestic services.[7] Others, such as Robert Hart, the customs inspector-general, fathered a second family in China.[8] Somewhat sheepishly, King confessed,

In those days the only "social" intercourse between Chinese and foreigners was conducted by women of the "Mui-tsai" class. In justice it must be recalled that the Chinese housekeeper often did a good deal to keep her temporary lord and master straight, especially in matters of drink, or tendency to stray off to less supervised and possibly dangerous-to-health pastures. Happily, all this is changed and gone forever. The number of marriageable girls of his own race all over China gives no excuse to a white man seeking a helpmeet to risk entangling alliances with native blood; but as a temporary measure in the old dark days—well, perhaps better not to hazard an opinion.[9]

Evidently, Manson did not avail himself of the "Jambarree spirit."[10] For eight years, he saved himself for his future wife. No doubt the many cases of syphilis and gonorrhea that he treated among merchant seamen and other Western men encouraged abstinence.[11] It is quite possible, too, that interracial sexual relations amounted to a needless expenditure of money and a diversion from his primary goal in China: to make money. And this goal he pursued with an impressive work ethic. After breakfast, Manson usually saw private Western clients on Kulangsu before he crossed the harbor to Amoy. Here he attended to the needs of patients at his dispensary and at the mission hospital while examining merchant seamen who arrived in port. Hiking and hunting excursions with male friends in the Fukien hinterland provided relief from the cares of his practice and apparently satisfied his emotional need for companionship (Figures 4 and 5).[12]

Although Manson denied himself sexual activity, he did not wish to deprive others of sexual relationships with Chinese women. In fact, in his capacity as a port surgeon, he called for the regulation of the casual sex trade in the port.[13] As Philippa Levine and others have shown, the regulation of prostitution was an established policy of the British imperial state after midcentury.[14] Alarmed by the spread of syphilis and gonorrhea among its personnel, imperial officials exerted control over the bodies of colonial women. Modeled on the Contagious Diseases Acts (1869) in Britain, which authorized the detainment and medical examination of women deemed by local authorities to be "common prostitutes," the registration and inspection of female sex workers became a regular policy

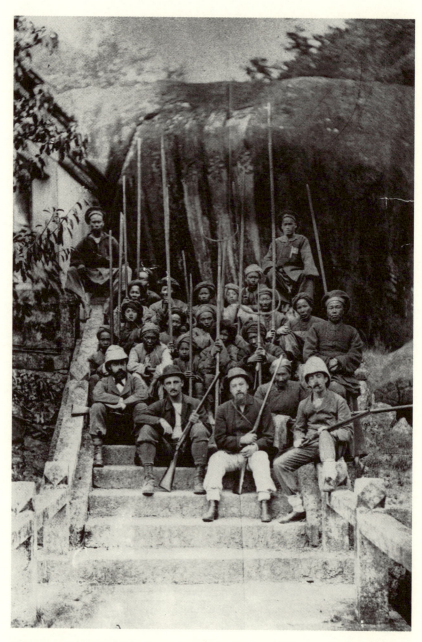

4. Manson as tiger hunter in 1874, Amoy, China. From Wellcome Institute Library, London. Manson is in front row, far left.

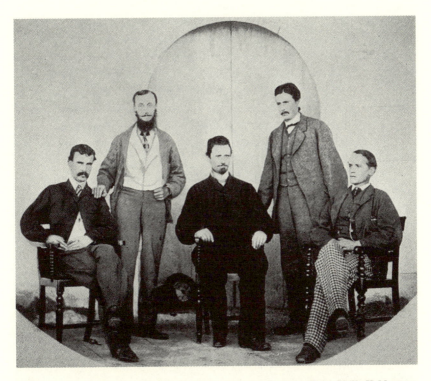

5. Manson (second from right) with friends in 1874, Amoy, China. From Philip H. Manson-Bahr, *Patrick Manson: The Father of Tropical Medicine* (London: Thomas Nelson, 1962).

in the second half of the nineteenth century in India, Hong Kong, Fiji, Gibraltar, and the Strait Settlements.[15]

In 1873, Manson announced that the time had come to introduce the Contagious Diseases Acts to Amoy. "It is painful to witness the progress and spread of so much mischief," Manson wrote in reference to the high numbers of infected crew members on the HBMS *Elk* in 1873, "wilful both on the part of the victim and on the part of those who might look after him better. It has been abundantly proved that syphilis can be stamped out by very simple measures." Mindful of the coalition of feminists and purity activists against the underlying sexual double standard of regulation in Britain, Manson anticipated little opposition in China. "These may meet with much opposition in many parts of Europe, but here, where on such subjects unglozed [*sic*] facts have made people more latitudinarian, there can be little to hinder the adoption of measures calculated to check and finally eradicate the disease."[16]

By the time Manson returned to Britain, he was very much in a marry-
ing mood. As a prosperous thirty-one-year-old, Manson sought the respect-
ability that only marriage to a European woman could confer in the foreign
settlement.[17] At the home of her uncle, he met Henrietta Isabella Thurburn, the
eighteen-year-old daughter of Captain J. P. Thurburn of the Royal Navy.[18] Although we do not possess the details of their courtship, it is likely that Manson made a favorable impression on Henrietta's parents. Besides being thir-
teen years older than Henrietta and a man of independent means, Manson was
available.

This was not a minor consideration. Raising a daughter for marriage was
uncertain in the best of times in the nineteenth century, but became even more
problematic after midcentury because of the rising surplus of women relative to
men. According to the 1871 census, women outnumbered men by nearly three-
quarters of a million. This imbalance, especially for the working classes, partly
reflected the effect of male emigration as well as protracted tours of duty in
the British army, navy, and merchant marine.[19] As Manson's own career reveals, the empire also attracted a significant number of middle-class males.
Middle-class women responded to these demographic trends: Some emigrated
in search of a husband, while others married imperial servants. The marriage
of Henrietta and Manson in December 1875, six months after they met, was
not so much predictable as representative of the demographic realities of marriage for men in the periphery and women in the metropole.[20] Their marriage,
like others, further domesticated the empire while relieving the metropolitan
marriage market of some pressure (Figure 6).

Manson and Elephantiasis in China

Before meeting Henrietta, Manson was a regular visitor to the reading room of
the British Museum. Here he devoted much of his time to studying two disease
conditions that he had encountered in Amoy: elephantiasis and lymph scrotum.
These diseases are not as distinctive as Manson and other investigators originally thought. They encompass a set of pathological conditions caused by the
presence of the *Filaria sanguinis hominis* worm in the human body. Despite
these and other diseases, its presence in humans is no accident. On the contrary, the body functions as a biological host in the development, or life cycle,
of this worm.

The means by which the *filaria* worm enters the human body presents
one of the most remarkable examples of adaptation in the animal kingdom.[21]

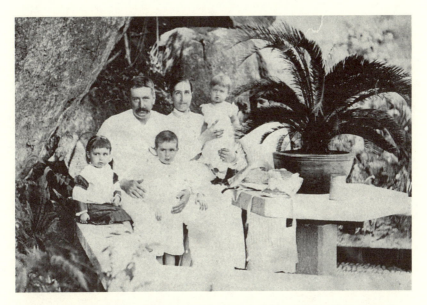

6. Manson with his wife, Henrietta Isabella, and their children, Amoy, China, 1881. From Wellcome Institute Library, London.

It begins in the evening, when the female *Culex fatigans* mosquito feeds on human blood. Observing the feeding habits of the mosquito, immature *filariae* or *microfilariae* surface in the peripheral bloodstream. In obeying her appetite, the mosquito serves a far more important imperative than simple pangs of hunger. To be sure, the blood meal provides the protein necessary for the development of the mosquito's progeny. It also furnishes a crucial means of locomotion for the *microfilariae*, which must leave the human body to continue its next stage of development. Ironically, the very protective sheath that envelops and protects the vulnerable ova in the bloodstream indefinitely arrests the developmental process. As it turns out, the evening meal of the mosquito rescues the ova from the ceaseless movement in and out of the peripheral bloodstream.

During this intermediary stage, which may last up to three weeks, the mosquito hosts numerous *microfilariae*. While some *microfilariae* succumb to the gastric juices of the mosquito, others do not. Shedding their sheaths, they grow into larvae (see Figure 7). These fortunate ones develop as they migrate through the abdominal and thoracic cavities of the mosquito. Their destination is the salivary glands of the proboscis, in which they reach their most advanced

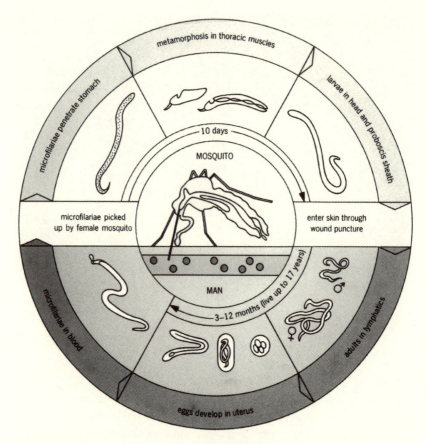

metamorphosis in thoracic muscles

larvae in head and proboscis sheath

microfilariae penetrate stomach

10 days

MOSQUITO

microfilariae picked
up by female mosquito

enter skin through
wound puncture

MAN

3–12 months (live up to 17 years)

microfilariae in blood

adults in lymphatics

eggs develop in uterus

7. Life cycle of lymphatic *filariae*. From Ralph Muller and John R. Baker, *Medical Parasitology* (London: Gower Medical Publications, 1990), 104.

development as larvae. From this point, their future development is dependent on the relentless hunger pangs of the female mosquito.

It is the subsequent blood meals that are responsible for spreading the infective larvae-stage worm among humans. The mosquito deposits the larvae not directly into the bloodstream but onto the skin in its saliva. When secreted on the skin, its saliva stimulates the flow of blood to the surface tissues. The larvae enter the body and are swept up in the swift currents of the body's fluids until they are deposited in a cavity. Obeying a survival instinct, they migrate toward the nutrient-rich lymphatic vessel network by burrowing through the tissues of the mesentery. Some form nodules and/or tumors along the lymphatic channels, while others become trapped in the lymph nodes and surrounding tissues.

In these sites, the larvae mature and become reproductively active. When fertilized, the viviparous female worms can produce thousands of immature *microfilariae*. The communication of nodules and tumors with the vascular system of the lymphatics enables a parent worm to disperse its progeny throughout the peripheral bloodstream, thereby maximizing their chances of being ingested by the hungry mosquito. Many die during the long and uncertain wait. Others may remain in the body as *microfilariae* for six months to two years. Adult worms have been known to live up to two years in the lymphatics.

In general, the presence of the *filariae* in the human body rarely leads to death. Neither death nor disease promotes the perpetuation of any parasite. Nevertheless, complications originate in the part of the body (namely, the lymphatic ducts, glands, and related circulatory system) that serves the interests of the *filariae*. This vascular network functions as an ideal source of sustenance and mode of dispersal of the *filaria*'s offspring. The pressure from tumors containing maturing worms or from the presence of too many ova can easily compromise the delicate walls of the lymphatics and cause the lymph and/or chyle to back up. In time, the volume of the fluid overwhelms the internal regulatory valves of the vessels, and this causes them to dilate. Arms and legs near compromised vessels may swell (hence the name elephantiasis) where the fluid has collected and takes on a jelly-like consistency. Permanent tumefaction is not the only result of the accumulation of lymph or chyle. The discharges of fluid from vesicles that form on the skin may deflate the bulk, as in the condition known as lymph scrotum. Or overflowing fluid from a vessel might seep into the renal tract and be expressed in the urine, causing chylous urine or tropical chyluria.

Manson encountered some of these very conditions shortly after joining the mission hospital in Amoy. *Filariasis* was endemic to South China, where a mobile population, together with a large reservoir of infected people, provided the ideal conditions for disease. Further, Chinese medicine lacked a therapeutic remedy, particularly in advanced cases. Although Western medical treatment was no more effective than Chinese medicine, Western surgery provided immediate relief from the discomfort caused by large tumors. When indigenous medicine failed, affected Chinese applied to the mission hospital because it offered an alternative and it was free.

Within his first year, Manson obtained enough experience with scrotal tumors to revise long-standing surgical practice. Surgeons in India as well as in Britain recommended either constricting the femoral artery to the affected region while excising the bulk or amputating the tumor along with the penis and testicles.[22] These practices reflected partly the belief that excessive tissue growth was due to an overabundant supply of blood, and partly the limitations of surgical intervention when death from blood loss and infection remained a distinct possibility.[23] While the former practice allowed the surgeon time to remove tumefied portions without excessive loss of blood, the risk of infection correspondingly increased. The latter practice reduced the loss of blood and infection, but at the expense of the penis and testicles.

Turning standard surgical practice on its head, Manson volunteered that "an increased circulation is more to be desired than an arrested or retarded one," lest the organs of the suprapubic region be deprived of a regular supply of blood. Constricting the blood supply at the neck of the tumor with a cord also ran the risk of damaging the integrity of the spermatic cords, testicles, and penis. Nor did pinning these organs by ligature necessarily produce better surgical outcomes, because this procedure did little to regulate the flow of blood to the tumor.[24]

Amputation provided a quick solution but increased the risk of excessive hemorrhaging. Manson warned, "A sudden escape of twenty ounces of blood is much more to be feared than the gradual loss of double that quantity." Faced with the retraction of the spermatic cord into the abdomen, the surgeon "will hesitate before he encounters the bleeding from two spermatic arteries and a dorsalis penis superadded to the supply of a fifty pound tumor," Manson added. Beyond the loss of blood, this procedure subjected the patient to shock and the contraction of the orifice following the cut of the urethra. Manson believed that "this operation should be discarded in every case, no matter how large the tumor."[25]

Manson's dissatisfaction with these practices spurred him to pioneer one of his own. It involved no new invasive instrument or technique, but instead concerned the preoperative preparation of the tumor. Manson recommended the placement of the tumor on a moveable board, attached to the operating table. When the tumor was elevated above the body, blood continued to flow to the affected region but gravity drained the superfluous blood from the tumor. This elevated position also furnished the surgeon with a better vantage point both to outline the bulk to be excised and to draw up the testicles, spermatic cord, and penis. Once these preoperative procedures were completed, the surgery itself consisted of excising the bulk and reconstructing a new scrotal sac from flaps of excess skin.[26]

While Manson was quite confident about correcting elephantiasis of the scrotum, he was less certain about another condition affecting the same region: lymph scrotum. Over two years, he encountered eight such cases. Typically, the inguinal lymphatic glands were dilated and the scrotum distended from the buildup of lymph fluid. Irregular discharges of lymph from vesicles relieved the scrotum of some of its bulk, but within days, the scrotum became "as big and cumbersome as before." This characteristic of the condition not only made surgical intervention of limited usefulness but also puzzled Manson regarding the precise pathological nature of the disease. "Why the lymph should not become organised into a tissue as in ordinary elephantiasis, when in the body, is the mystery of the disease. Perhaps some explanation of this may be afforded by the abscess which in most instances precedes the development of the vesicles, or there may be some radical difference between this and the ordinary form of elephantiasis, rendering this 'lymph-scrotum' a disease sui generis."[27]

It was this mystery which spurred Manson to survey the literature on the diseases of the suprapubic region at the library of the British Museum. Here, however, Manson did not find confirmation of the specificity of lymph scrotum as a disease. Instead, he found a wider framework for understanding the diseases he encountered in China. The published work of several Anglo-Indian investigators persuaded Manson to see the compromised lymphatic system as the generic seat of a group of distinctive disease conditions: lymph scrotum, elephantiasis, and tropical chyluria. They also disabused him of the idea of "malarial fever" as the etiological agent of disease. This displacement of an environmental cause created a space for Manson's acceptance of the *filaria* worm as the presumptive agent of disease for the three hitherto distinct conditions.

Discovering the Filaria Sanguinis Hominis *Worm in London*

The image of Manson poring over medical journals at the British Museum is an ambiguous one. On the one hand, it underscores his continuing marginality within the metropolitan profession. The reciprocity provision of the 1858 Medical Act technically placed Manson's medical degree from Aberdeen University on the same footing as qualifications from the London-based Royal Colleges of Surgeons or Physicians. A qualification from either institution would not have improved his prospects as a port officer or as a private practitioner in China. Yet in Britain, such qualifications remained essential for public positions ranging from the poor law medical services to the leading metropolitan hospitals. Membership also conferred the right to use the well-endowed libraries of the Royal Colleges. Manson did not need to be told that he was an outsider. He had made the decision to be one at the beginning of his career.

On the other hand, the Colleges were notoriously indifferent to the practice of medicine in the empire. Before the Bengal branch of the British Medical Association, Dr. Joseph Fayrer, of the Bengal Army, volunteered, "You will have difficulty in adducing even a causal reference, in any of the standard works in Britain professing to treat exhaustively of their respective subjects, to the authority, practice or opinion of one Indian surgeon." [28] Alexander Faulkner, of the Bombay Medical Service, informed readers of the *British Medical Journal* that "its admirable contemporary, the Indian Medical Gazette, is characterized by its absence in most of the medical libraries in England. I feel sure that the Indian Medical Gazette only requires to be known, and its perusal would be appreciated by the frequenters of these libraries, many of whom are interested in the professional work carried out in and peculiar to India." [29]

For Manson's interest in the diseases of the lymphatics, few metropolitan medical libraries could rival the range of the library of the British Museum. In all but name, this library was an imperial institution. It served as a repository of the research activities of the far-flung British empire, especially British India.[30] In the wake of the Mutiny in 1857, British India boasted one of the largest medical communities in the empire outside Britain.[31] Although marginalized from the metropolitan profession, imperial doctors created their own institutions. These included the Medical and Physical Society of Bombay, the Lahore Medical Club, the Medical and Physical Society of Haiderbad, and the Bengal Branch of the British Medical Association. A far larger number followed Anglo-Indian professional affairs through their own medical press, which included the *Indian Annals of Medicine*, *Indian Medical Gazette*, *Transactions of the Medical and Physical Society of Bombay*, *Journal of the Madras Medical Society*, and *Transactions of the Medical and Physical Society of Calcutta*.[32]

Medical knowledge in India was anything but static.[33] This professional culture created a context for the exploration of the pathology and etiology of *filariasis*. Elephantiasis was familiar to practitioners, particularly in the lower provinces of Bengal and along the Malabar coast of Madras, where the disease was endemic. There was no settled consensus about the seat of the disease. Some viewed it as a result of the inflammation of the veins; others believed the cause to be the inflammation of the lymphatics. In 1861, H. Vandyke Carter, a member of the Bombay Medical Service and professor of anatomy and physiology at the Bombay Medical School, recast the discussion altogether.[34] In a discussion of chylous urine, Carter showed the relationship of the varicose or dilated condition of the lymphatics to disease and related this condition to other diseases, including elephantiasis and lymph scrotum.[35]

For Manson, Carter's article raised as many questions as answers. On the one hand, he offered validation for Manson's suggestion that lymph scrotum was a disease located in the varicose condition of the lymphatics. On the other hand, Carter's generic pathological seat for elephantiasis, chylous urine, and lymph scrotum raised a further question: Was there a generic etiological cause? By confining himself to the pathology of *varix lymphaticus*, Carter sidestepped this question altogether. But as Manson's reading journal records, this question was one that interested other Anglo-Indian investigators. At issue was whether elephantiasis was caused by malarial fever or not.

For practitioners in the tropical world, malarial fever served as the default category for disease. As such, it mirrored the possibilities and limitations of the representation of disease. From the clinical perspective, the term *malaria* referred to the presentation of a familiar set of signs of disease, such as the onset of fever or the enlargement of the spleen. From the epidemiological perspective, the association of illness and disease with the tropical world transformed the very environment into an etiological agent. In the absence of a specific causal agent, practitioners purported to find malarial poisons virtually everywhere in the tropical environment—in hot and cool climates, in deserts and lush landscapes, and in undeveloped and developed regions.[36]

As a type of figurative language for disease, then, malarial fever collapsed the clinical and epidemiological perspective. However, this very rhetorical function generated as much conflict as consensus among practitioners. It could not completely mask the variety of experience or reconcile it with disease. Was fever the primary cause or a secondary concomitant of disease? This question, as it applied to elephantiasis, exposed the inherently unstable nature of disease classification while simultaneously creating the possibility for the consideration of alternative pathogens.

Edward John Waring, a surgeon in the Madras Medical Service and physician to the rajah of Travancore, deduced that malarial fever caused localized swelling. In his article in the *Indian Annals of Medical Science*, he reported this sequence in 224 out of 226 cases under his care. Patient observations, collected by native subordinates and by Dr. Pringle of the Cochin Civil Service, confirmed this causal relationship. Out of 658 designated cases, Waring wrote that "458, or 70 per cent, attributed [the disease] to fever; and what more natural than they should do so, seeing that febrile attack had been the immediate precursor of the enlargement of limb?"[37]

Waring's conclusion elicited a range of opinion. Writing in the *Transactions of the Medical and Physical Society of Bombay*, George Ballingall, a member of the Bombay Medical Service, doubted a causal relationship between fever and localized swelling: "In cases which have fallen under my own observation I have not observed any regularity as to the accession of inflammation."[38] Charles Morehead disagreed with his colleague: "I still retain the opinion . . .

that the disease is endemic, the fever primary, and the deposit secondary—just as the albuminous deposits in the liver and spleen are secondary on recurring intermittent fever." [39]

For others, the clinical signs of elephantiasis did not conform to those of malarial disease—at least, as they understood it. Civil surgeon Francis Day, in his article on "Cochin leg," which appeared in the *Madras Quarterly Journal of Medical Science*, drew a sharp distinction between the clinical presentations of the two conditions.

The paroxysms of elephantoid fever always come on daily like quotidians, never as tertians, or quartans, and are unchecked by antiperiodics: the cold stage is often excessive: headache peculiar, delirium, rare in agues, is here frequent and persistent for days: pulse slightly altered; constipation nearly invariable: buboes, absent in agues, here present: feverish attacks violent, without corresponding permanent constitutional injury: effusions become organized, and added to in each succeeding attack: complications such as are commonly perceived intermittent, are also absent: no coughs, dysenteries, nor diarrhoeas, except in a few cases which are generally progressing favourably.[40]

Vincent Richards, civil medical officer of Balasore, agreed. In northern Orissa, Richards reported that fever usually followed the onset of local swelling. Although he confirmed the regular presence of fever in most clinical cases, he doubted its inherent malarial character. "With all due deference to those who hold a contrary opinion, I think too little is known of the relative causes and effects of malaria, to warrant our concluding that, because paroxysms of a fever are regular, it follows that they depend upon one combination of causes." [41]

This dispute about the nature of elephantiasis in India was not lost on Manson. Before returning to Britain, he had ascribed scrotal disease to "malarial influence" or "malaria fever." Like other European practitioners, he customized his malarial cause even though his cases of elephantiasis and lymph scrotum did not consistently conform to the characteristics of malarial disease, that is, the presence of fever and/or an enlarged spleen. By simply invoking the tropical environment, Manson explained away these anomalies. "Such cases at first sight appear to militate against the hypothesis we have expressed," Manson conceded, "but they may receive an explanation similar to that applicable to those instances of enlargement of the spleen, neither accompanied nor preceded by ague, but depending on malaria cachexia, the result of life from childhood in a malarious atmosphere, and descent from parents long the subjects of malarious disease. Both diseases have the same origin, and both present the same variations in development and progress." [42]

Manson quickly came to appreciate the inadequacy of malarial fever as an etiological agent. When summarizing Day's views on the cause of elephantiasis, he rhetorically asked, "Is it malarious and like enlarged spleen does the local disease depend on poison?" He then answered no.[43] But the discrediting of malarial fever as etiological cause simply made the question that Carter's article raised all the more pressing, namely, what caused the lymphatics to dilate? It was at this point that Manson learned about the discovery of the coexistence of immature *filariae* worms or *microfilariae* in several chylous cases from Timothy R. Lewis, a surgeon in the British army who served under the sanitary commissioner with the government of India, in a series of articles in the *Indian Medical Gazette*.[44]

In March 1870, Lewis detected "delicate filaments" when examining the milky discharge from a chylous case under the microscope. Initially, he regarded these forms as little more than fungus associated with urine. But their tendency to "coil and uncoil themselves" soon convinced Lewis that they were in fact living forms. Aided by a network of colleagues at native hospitals, Lewis detected immature worms in the urine of twenty cases, as well as in the blood of four cases, over the next two years. The coexistence of these worms with urinary disease led Lewis to suggest a causal relationship.

[Their presence] may lead to local stoppages in the flow of the nutritive fluids and to rupture of the extremely delicate walls of the capillaries, lacteal or lymphatics. The extreme activity of the Filariae, especially should a bundle of them accumulate in one particular spot, would doubtless materially aid in giving rise to rupture—for, as is well known, the walls of these channels are extremely delicate, those of the lymphatic system being especially so. The resulting phenomena, such as the escape of the nutritive fluid and of the *Filariae* contained within the ruptured channel into the excretory ducts belonging to the part, appears to me to be so simple a procedure that to dilate on its mechanisms would be quite superfluous.[45]

Lewis's report intrigued Surgeon K. McLeod, editor of the *Indian Medical Gazette*. Based on several case histories that exhibited two or more conditions, McLeod declared "an unquestional [*sic*] pathological alliance between the various morbid conditions which have been referred to, viz. chyluria, chylous, and lymphous discharges from the skin, elephantiasis and hydrocele, points to the lymphatic vessels and glands as being the substratum of these forms of morbid nutrition." Yet, as promising as McLeod found Lewis's discovery, he called for further research. "The natural history of the *filariae* which Dr. Lewis has discovered has still to be worked out, and the pathogenesis of these various morbid states evolved."[46]

The matter of the life cycle of the *filaria* was critical to the overall integrity of Lewis's discovery. Lewis grounded a causal pathological relationship between the *filaria* worm and human disease based on a host-parasite relationship. This latter relationship explained disease as a product not of chance or even environment but of the interdependence of two organisms. The presence of ova in the bloodstream implied that an active parent worm existed and, by extension, that the *filaria* was adapted to live in the human body unharmed.[47] Demonstrating this adaptive relationship, however, was another matter. The life cycle of the worm was hardly known. Lewis had identified neither the adult nor the larval form of the parasite. At the time of his first report, he could only infer that the bloodstream was the temporary "home" of the *microfilariae* based on its arrested development while inside the protective sheath.[48]

In the meantime, Lewis continued his investigations into the life cycle of the *filaria*. Unable to procure human bodies to search for the adult or parent of the *microfilaria*, he turned to dogs in hopes of shedding comparative light on the human *filaria*. The postmortem examination of dogs infected with *F. sanguinolenta* revealed the tissue damage associated with its migratory activity. Tumors and nodules, containing adults and immature worms, respectively, were embedded in the walls of the thoracic aorta and along the esophagus tract. In turn, Lewis found a correspondence between the presence of ova in the peripheral blood of living dogs and the network of tunnels through which the orifices of the nodules and tumors communicated with the aorta. By this means, adult worms dispersed their offspring throughout the body by way of the peripheral bloodstream.[49]

Beyond identifying the adult worm and its offspring, Lewis was unable to detect any free embryos—that is, those liberated from the ova shell—in the bloodstream. Their detection, at least in theory, would have completed the life cycle of the worm from ovum to adult. But, rather than undermining Lewis's confidence in a biological relationship between the *filaria* worm and the dog, the absence of free embryos reinforced it. According to the principle of alternative generation, their absence was not at all surprising. As proposed by Danish naturalist Johannes Japetus Steenstrup in 1842 and extended by continental naturalists by midcentury, under this principle the offspring of a parasite not only assumed an appearance that was dissimilar from that of its parent but also developed in more than one host before assuming the appearance of the adult.[50] This principle informs Lewis's description of the next stage of development of the embryo and his experimental cultivation of ova.

Lewis's sketch of the next stage of the embryo was an invention. It only approximated a developmental middle point between the adult worm and its undeveloped ova, when "the ova or liberated embryos of the *Filaria sanguino-lenta* find their way in a 'host' or other medium suitable for their development during the larval stage—a stage in their development carried on, possibly, to the extent of providing the embryo with some kind of oral armature and a differentiated intestinal tube [*sic*]." From this point, the future of the embryo depends on its being ingested by its primary host. "Having acquired this stage of growth the further progress of the parasite is dependent on its being swallowed by some such animal as the dog, to the mucous lining of whose oesophagus it attaches itself, then penetrating the muscular tissue of this tube and remaining there or working its way still further until it reaches the tissues of the thoracic aorta, or some other place suitable to its growth and development." [51]

To test this inference, Lewis tried to cultivate ova of the *F. sanguinolenta* in the external environment and in animals that dogs might eat. But without a more specific basis for narrowing the range of intermediary host-candidates, these experiments were doomed to fail. "I have made numerous attempts at bringing the embryos to maturity; by means of moist earth; by feeding cockroaches with bread soaked in fluid containing ova; by introducing ova into the stomach and peritoneal cavity of frogs, etc., but have not yet succeeded—the ova and their contained embryos being, from a week to a fortnight afterwards, detected in the bodies of the animals without having undergone any apparent change." [52]

In February 1875, the *Indian Medical Gazette* reviewed Lewis's 1874 report, which also appeared in the *Indian Annals of Medical Science*. For his part, McLeod balanced his enthusiasm for Lewis's discovery against the circumstantial nature of the research record. Although he doubted that canine *filaria* required a further stage outside its primary host, McLeod agreed that *Filaria sanguinolenta* "is the parent of the brood of immature embryo constituting the haematozoa in the dog" and that "the development of the latter takes place in some tissue of the dog." McLeod still tempered the inferences that could legitimately be drawn from comparative research: "If conclusions can be drawn from analogy in such matters it would seem probable that the human being infested by haematozoa must harbor a parent worm in some tissue or organ; but no such worm has as yet been discovered." [53] Similarly, the speculative role of *filaria* in causing disease in humans, while suggestive, nevertheless proved to be inconclusive.[54] "These speculations are exceedingly ingenious, and, in the view of the ascertained facts regarding canine haematozoa, very probable; but their demonstration as positive fact is still wanting." [55]

Unlike McLeod, with his guarded encouragement, Manson entertained few doubts about the role of the *filaria* worm in human disease.[56] Even though he formed his opinions from secondary sources, it made perfect sense to him. As a matter of fact, months before returning to China, Manson prepared a short report of his literature survey on *filaria* disease for his colleagues in the customs service. Modeling his report on the transformation of his own thinking, Manson framed the etiological significance of the *filaria* worm first by foregrounding the generic pathological seat of elephantiasis, lymph scrotum, and chyluria in the dilated lymphatics. From here, he posed the same question that Carter's research had raised: "What then is the cause of this condition?"[57]

Manson abandoned malarial fever as the cause of localized swelling. Fever represented, at most, a secondary effect of the "distension of the lymphatics." He now attributed disease to the obstruction of nutritive fluids in the lymphatics vessel caused by the activity of the worm.

The calibre of the lymphatics, and even of the thoracic duct, is very small, and could easily be obstructed by a minute body. In consequence of this interference to the progress upwards of the lymph, there is accumulation on the distal side of the stoppage, dilation of lymphatics, perhaps rupture in parts where their walls are very thin or superficial as in the scrotum (lymph scrotum), or bladder (chyluria), or perhaps only stasis and accumulation of lymph materials which undergo a certain amount of organisation (elephantiasis).[58]

The life cycle of the worm in the body, Manson added, illuminated the particular timing of the manifestation of disease itself.

After a time the parent nematode dies or escapes; the tumour that enclosed it is absorbed or disintegrated; the lymph channel again becomes patent, its circulation is renewed, and the chyle disappears from the urine, the scrotum no longer discharges, or the elephantiasis ceases to increase. Other nematodes progress in their development (in the thoracic aorta of the same dog they may be found in all stages of development); the lymph channel is again obstructed (perhaps in a different place, producing the appearance of metastasis, a thing well known to happen in elephantoid disease), there is a fresh attack of chyluria, lymph scrotum or elephantiasis.[59]

Manson's interest in *filariasis* did not end with this report. The report marked the beginning of Manson's future research. Up to this point, no one had identified the adult worm, much less described the development of the *microfilariae* outside the bloodstream. For a port surgeon, research did not offer any rewards. Instead, for Manson as for other imperial doctors, research provided a cultural vehicle to transcend the geographical marginality of the periphery by participating in a far-flung community of investigators engaged in producing knowledge about the empire. Why else did Manson communicate the results of his survey of the literature on *filariasis* to the *Medical Times and Gazette* before returning to China?[60] Or, for that matter, why did he forward copies of his customs reports on scrotal disease to the leading metropolitan specialists on the diseases of the skin and pubic region?[61]

By transforming local knowledge into categories of European medical science, investigators in the empire did not simply engage in the rudimentary collection of information as directed from the metropole. Rather, they participated as active agents in the constitution of British medicine as imperial medicine. William Aitken, the author of one of Manson's medical reference books, said as much when he exhorted imperial doctors to make the most of their opportunities for research on the relationship of parasites to diseases.[62]

The relative connection which these circumstances have to one another have scarcely yet attracted the attention of pathologists, human or comparative. Here, indeed, is a wide field for investigation—a territory yet unexplored. The medical service of Her Majesty's British and Indian armies gives golden chances for observations, if the chances are seized at the moment, and the observations connected with facts already known.[63]

Isolating the Mosquito as "Nurse"

Once Manson had returned to Amoy, mundane matters shaped his research orientation. It was difficult to make time in an already long work day, and human bodies for postmortem examinations were difficult to obtain. The Chinese prohibition against disturbing the bodies of the dead precluded in short order the search for the adult representative of the *filaria*, lodged deep in the tissue cavities of the body. "The privilege," Manson wrote in reference to the only postmortem examination he conducted, "had to be paid for, and was hampered with the condition that the widow should be present to see that no part of the body was removed. Besides it had to be made secretly with closed doors, quickly, and in the room the man died in, a place hardly big enough to turn in. The light was very bad and the heat overpowering. So from this unfortunate combination of circumstances the examination was far from thorough or satisfactory, and did not result, as I hoped, in the discovery of the parent worm."[64]

The lack of human subjects did not discourage Manson, however. Following Lewis's example, he turned to the comparative study of canine *filaria*.[65] Dogs were plentiful in the foreign settlement, including strays, lame hunting dogs, and house pets. From these dogs, Manson studied *Filariae immitis* and *Filariae sanguinolentae*, two blood worms native to China and well known to naturalists. Even though Manson's study shed little new light on these worms, the exercise was beneficial. Searching for and studying these worms improved his microscopic skills as well as his understanding of the anatomy and physiology of the *filaria* species. This study, too, enabled Manson to evaluate the structural damage caused by the activity of adult worms and offspring in their hosts.

Needless to say, comparative research did not advance Manson's primary interest, namely, identifying the adult worm in the human body. Just as Manson adjusted his research interest in response to the availability of human bodies, the chance detection of the *microfilariae* in the blood opened up a new avenue of research. In an addendum to his canine *filaria* study, Manson indicated the import of the presence of *microfilariae* in a scrotal case: "I am thus enabled to state positively that elephantiasis Arabum is a parasitic disease and to establish on solid and incontrovertible grounds, what in a former report I conjectured was the true pathology of this puzzling affection." [66]

From this point, Manson rapidly turned his attention from the pathology to the epidemiology of *filaria* disease. By revealing the distribution of the parasite in the population served by the mission hospital, Manson hoped to fortify the case for a causal relationship between parasite and human disease. [67] Practically, it was an easy decision to make. As physician to the hospital, Manson had virtually unlimited access to the residents of Amoy and environs who sought medical attention. The ready availability of hospital assistants enabled Manson to delegate the time-consuming task of searching microscopically for the *microfilariae* in blood smears while servicing his large practice. [68]

Over the course of several months, Manson and his assistants examined the blood of some 670 subjects. They detected *microfilariae* in sixty-two patients, or 9.2 percent of those who applied to the hospital for treatment but did not exhibit the symptoms of *filaria* disease. The frequency of the *microfilariae* suggested that its presence in the human body was more than an accident. The coexistence of the *microfilariae* in cases with multiple disease conditions—that is, elephantiasis and allied disease cases—was even more telling: 58 percent in elephantiasis and lymph scrotum combined with tropical chyluria and 25.8 percent in cases that exhibited inflamed scrota and fever. To Manson, the conclusion was inescapable: "Mere coincidence will not account for the frequent, and in some forms of the disease almost invariable, association of the parasite and the disease; they can only stand to each other in the relation of cause and consequence." [69]

Manson's study did not end here. The presence of *microfilariae* in the population and its coexistence with disease presented compelling circumstantial evidence of a causal relationship. Since no known parasite completed its entire life cycle in a single human host, Manson had to explain how the *micro-filariae* entered and left the body. Without this critical link in the life cycle of the parasite, the presence of the *filariae* in the human body could still be seen, at best, as associated with disease or, at worst, accidental. For Manson, the female *Culex fatigans* mosquito as the intermediary host proved to be the missing piece in the puzzle.

Although Manson is credited with isolating the mosquito, he did not work alone. Lewis's research provided valuable markers for Manson, particularly as the orientation of his investigation into *filariasis* changed. Well before he detected the *microfilariae* for himself in 1876, Manson gave little attention to Lewis's cultivation experiments regarding the future life cycle of canine *filariae* ova and embryos. By his own admission, Manson did not know how to search for the *microfilaria* microscopically.[70] But once Manson turned to the epidemiology of *filaria* disease in Amoy, Lewis's inference about the blood as the "temporary home" of the *microfilariae* assumed a much more important place in his thinking. Although Lewis appears to have made no search for the intermediary host of the *microfilariae* outside their primary host, he did so a year later, analogously, in his comparative study of canine *filaria*.

As it turned out, Lewis's ova and embryo cultivation trials proved to be more valuable to Manson as failures. These failed experiments induced Manson to contemplate a more specialized intermediary host than Lewis's seemingly random host-candidates. Since *microfilariae* existed in the bloodstream for a brief period, Manson surmised that the "privilege" of hosting it was "confined to a very limited number of animals—the bloodsuckers." These included "fleas, lice, bugs, leeches, mosquitos, and sandflies." By deduction, Manson pared down the number of host-candidates further by correlating the geographical distribution of the parasite in tropical regions of the world with the incidence of the disease. "But as the parasite is confined to a limited area of the earth's surface it is more than likely that this friend of the filaria has a corresponding and limited distribution. Fleas, lice, bugs, leeches, as they are found pretty well all over the world, must therefore be excluded."[71]

Manson quickly rigged a human-biting experiment to test this hypothesis. Using his position at the hospital, he appropriated the body of Hin-Lo, one of his patients. While Hin-Lo was sleeping in a screened compartment in a crude shack, Manson allowed wild mosquitoes to feed on the patient. "After [Hin-Lo] had gone to bed a light was placed beside him, and the door of the mosquito-house kept open for half an hour. In this way many mosquitoes entered the 'house'; the light was then put out, and the door closed," Manson recalled. In the morning, Manson's assistant disabled the satiated mosquitoes that covered the walls with a puff of tobacco smoke before transferring them to ventilated glass phials. Manson examined the "stomach" contents of these mosquitoes, staggered over a week.[72]

From his observations, Manson described the development of the *microfilaria* from "a simple structureless animal" to a "being otherwise suited for an independent existence after it left."[73] Measuring it against our contemporary knowledge, historians have marvelled at Manson's close approximation of the intermediary stage.[74] Once the mosquito ingests *microfilariae*, the embryos lose their sheaths just as Manson reported. Over the next four to seventeen hours, they penetrate the lining of the abdomen en route to the thoracic muscles. After seven to ten days in the thoracic cavity, the larvae lose their tails and assume a sausage shape. The body cavities and intestinal canal, which Manson accurately described, become visible, as does the outline of the genitalia. From this point, Manson's narrative faltered. The larvae do not pass out of the mosquito into water before being passively ingested by humans. Instead, they remain for another week or more. During this period, they achieve their maximum size while migrating to the labella in preparation for injection into the human bloodstream.[75]

What is even more remarkable is how Manson could have arrived at this narrative of development with an experiment so riddled with flaws. Not only did Manson conduct just one feeding experiment but the mosquitoes that fed on Hin-Lo were wild. Nor did Manson inspect the abdominal and thoracic cavities of mosquitoes systematically when searching for the ingested *microfilariae*. Instead, he commingled the viscera, which he described as an undifferentiated "stomach."[76] These defects in experimental practice may, to be sure, reflect an inexperienced investigator. They also suggest the degree to which Manson's desire to fortify the case for a causal relationship between the *filaria* and disease prevented him from recognizing anomalies in his results. Neither the presence of *filariae* of varying sizes early in the developmental cycle nor their paucity in the latter stage suggested that the mosquito required more than one blood meal, nor did he see the need for a second feeding experiment to verify his narrative of development.

Manson's use of rhetoric was essential in the representation of his observations as a linear narrative of biological change. By organizing his observations into three arbitrary stages of development, Manson effectively elided over the multiple and rapidly changing forms.[77] Stage one, which required thirty-six hours, commenced when the embryos entered the mosquito. After several hours, the sheath that enveloped the embryo while it was in the human bloodstream separated from the body. Surface transverse markings became visible.

Toward the end of the first stage, Manson recognized oral movements, more distinctive striation, and the complete separation of the sheath.[78]

The second, or chrysalis, stage overlapped the first. Body and oral movements ceased, though the tail continued to flex and extend. By the end of the third day, the embryo was broader in width and shorter, but the tail retained its original sharp outline. Development was most noticeable in the large central cells that massed in the center of the body cavity, where Manson detected a faint line from the oral aperture to the caudal extremity, prefiguring the alimentary canal.[79]

After the fourth day, Manson had difficulty in obtaining living specimens from his mosquitoes.[80] He managed to find four four-day-old *filariae* from among several hundred mosquitoes at the commencement of the third and final stage. Their presence among less developed embryos in a single mosquito confirmed their relationship to each other.[81] At this stage, the tail shrank to a "stump" while the body of the embryo grew in length and width; its movement became "brisker"; the oral aperture became more distinct, as did the once-faint line of the alimentary canal, which now linked it to an unmistakable caudal extremity.[82] Manson also reported the appearance of a new structure near the caudal extremity, crowned with three or four papillae, which concluded stage three.

There is no question that Manson observed change in the *filaria* while it was in the mosquito over the course of a week. But Manson's interpretation of change was driven not so much by induction as by his conviction that the mosquito was the intermediary host. The third stage, like the other two, was little more than a fiction, one that concealed the arbitrary nature of Manson's representation of *filaria* development. The third stage was "final" not least because the mosquito's death from starvation terminated *filaria* growth. It, too, anticipated the future history of the *filaria* in water while masking the fact that Manson's narrative of development was based on a single, unverified feeding experiment.

At this, presumably the final stage of the filaria's existence in the mosquito, it becomes endowed with marvellous power and activity. It rushes about the field forcing obstacles aside, moving indifferently after either end, and appears quite at home and in no way inconvenienced by the water it has just been immersed in. This formidable looking animal is undoubtedly the Filaria sanguinis hominis equipped for independent life and ready to quit its nurse the mosquito.[83]

The speculative "water" phrase served a rhetorical purpose as well. As a medium of transmission, it bridged the life of the *filaria* between the primary and intermediary hosts. "There can be little doubt as to the subsequent history of the filaria; or that escaping into the water in which the mosquito died, it is through the medium of this fluid brought into contact with the tissues of man, and then either piercing the integuments, or, what is more probable, being swallowed, it works its way through the alimentary canal to its final resting place," Manson insisted. From this point, the life cycle is completed. "Arrived there its development is perfected, fecundation is effected, and finally the embryo filariae we meet with in the blood are discharged in successive swarms and in countless numbers." [84]

*   *   *

Much like his career, Manson's interest in *filariasis* was a product of the dialectical relationship between the imperial metropole and its periphery. Facilitating this relationship were furloughs for imperial servants and imperial cultural institutions such as the library of the British Museum. By virtue of its power to collect and organize knowledge from the periphery, the library mediated the production of imperial knowledge. As an archive of the empire, the library provided a space for Manson to situate the distinctive diseases that he encountered in China in a wider context. Here Manson adjusted his understanding of the etiology of *filaria* disease based on the work of Anglo-Indian investigators, especially Timothy R. Lewis. By the end of his furlough, Manson abandoned malarial fever as the cause of elephantiasis and lymph scrotum. Thereafter, he regarded these and other conditions as products of the intersection of the life cycle of the *filaria* worm with humans.

Yet this very dialectic between the metropole and the periphery made the production of imperial knowledge an inherently political enterprise. Where did the authority to define and legitimize imperial knowledge originate? In the metropole or in the periphery? This was not an idle question, particularly for imperial doctors. Their very social, not to mention geographical, marginality within British society as imperial servants placed them in a dependent position vis-à-vis metropolitan investigators. Manson was clearly sensitive to the underlying social politics of imperial science. Otherwise, he would not have solicited the endorsement of Timothy R. Lewis of Calcutta as well as that of Thomas B. Cobbold, a London-based natural scientist, concerning his discovery.

The timing of Manson's letters turned out to be propitious. For two years, Lewis and Cobbold had been embroiled in a contentious dispute in the medical press regarding the priority of discovery of the embryo and adult representative of the *filaria* worm. Each was motivated by the desire to be associated

with the discovery of the different stages of the first known human blood parasite. But this dispute was no less a power struggle between workers, one in
the metropole and one in the periphery, over the authority to define scientific
knowledge about the empire. As the next chapter will show, this dispute helped
to transform Manson's flawed narrative of the intermediary stage of the *filaria*
worm into a normative part of its life cycle.

3

The Rhetoric and Politics of Discovery

THE metropolitan medical press played a critical role in constructing knowledge about the empire. From time to time imperial doctors, to be sure, complained about the profession's indifference to medicine in the empire.[1] But it would be misleading to suggest that the Victorian medical press was indifferent either to the empire or to imperial doctors. On the contrary, the *Lancet*, the *British Medical Journal*, and the *Medical Times and Gazette*, to name a few, foregrounded the empire in a number of formats.[2] They regularly published student examination results for the Army Medical School at Netley and the Naval Medical School at Haslar and promotion lists for the state services, that is, the Army, Indian, and Naval Medical Services. Editorials roundly deplored the social subordination of medical professionals in the state services and colonial services of the dependent empire. The correspondence pages carried advertisements for private practices and printed requests for information about prospects in the self-governing colonies of white settlement. Original articles on diseases and special features on epidemics in the empire formed part of the staple coverage on preventive medicine and public health. Finally, short notices on the activities of professional societies as well as book reviews kept the empire before the profession.

The coverage of the empire had cultural consequences for British medicine: It enmeshed the metropolitan profession, as much as it did practitioners in the empire, in the processes of imperialism. The rhetorical accessibility of the empire diminished the distance between practitioners in the metropole and in the periphery while transforming the metropolitan medical press into a medium of imperial medicine. Ideologically, the representation of indigenous practices as backward and of the periphery as an alternative disease space did more than simply register the European encounter with alien environments and systems of medicine. It helped to consolidate the image of Britain as a healthy and advanced society and British medicine as a force for progress and a symbol of modernity.

However, it would be equally misleading to suggest that the process of making imperial knowledge was a harmonious one. The very function of the press politicized the process. By expediting the circulation of news and information about the periphery, metropolitan publicity increased, rather than diminished, the conflict over the priority of discovery. Underlying these disputes were the social tensions between workers in the empire and those at home. Who was best qualified to authorize or authenticate new knowledge? Was it the specialist in the periphery or the one in the metropole? The former, who emigrated for better prospects, or the latter, who made his way in London?

It should not come as a surprise that conflict defined the discovery of the different stages of the life cycle of the *Filaria sanguinis hominis* worm, the only known parasite adapted to exist in the human bloodstream. The discovery of the *filaria* worm was a considerable novelty and source of constant friction between Thomas S. Cobbold, a leading natural scientist based in London, and Timothy R. Lewis, a surgeon in the British army in India (Figure 8). The pages of the medical press not only enabled Cobbold and Lewis to transcend geography in the pursuit of their common interests but also provided each with a medium to secure scientific credit for the identification of the immature and adult stages of the *filaria* worm. Over several years, their dispute received regular coverage in one format or another, including original communications, lead articles, research notices, reports on medical societies, letters to the editor, and book reviews.

The publicized conflict between Cobbold and Lewis led to Manson's discovery of the mosquito as intermediary host of the *filaria* worm by generating an audience for its reception. Writing from China, Manson solicited the endorsement of Cobbold and Lewis, who had previously feuded over credit for the discovery of the adult stage. They arrived at opposing views about the significance of Manson's research. Cobbold announced the discovery of the intermediary host based on Manson's account and slide preparations of *filaria* development. After failing to verify experimentally the development of the larval stage as Manson reported, Lewis published a skeptical report within months after Cobbold's announcement. While these conflicting conclusions raised doubts about the credibility of Manson's discovery, they nonetheless created a rhetorical space for its validation. As this chapter will show, Manson and the mosquito prevailed not because of the explanatory power of experimental science alone but in concert with the effective use of metropolitan publicity.

What's in a Name?

Thomas S. Cobbold was one of the *new men* of Victorian natural science. These men were from the broadly defined middle classes, often university educated, and typically trained as medical professionals. The vast, uncharted fields of botany, geology, and zoology fired their imaginations. Mastering the natural world through knowledge offered a self-affirming ideology for men who sought to shape their own destinies and to consolidate their positions as public scientists in society. But transforming their passions into careers was a decidedly uncertain venture. There were few remunerative positions. Success, therefore, required not only an inquiring mind but also a propensity for self-promotion.

After completing his medical degree at Edinburgh University in 1851, Cob-

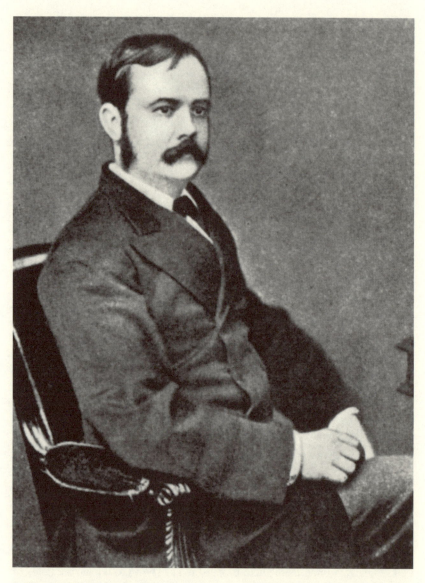

8. Timothy Richard Lewis (1841–86) (above) and Thomas Spencer Cobbold (1828–86). From John D. Comrie, *History of Scottish Medicine*, 2 vols. (London: Baillière, Tindall and Cox, 1932), 2:780.

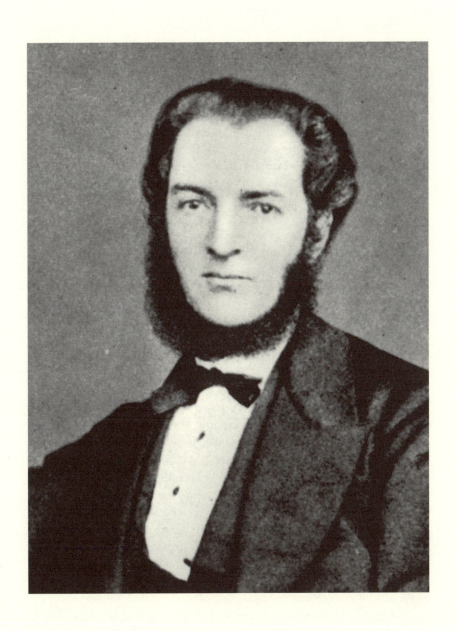

bold served as curator to the University Anatomical Museum. Six years later, he moved to London. Here he patched together a living by lecturing on botany at St. Mary's Hospital and on comparative anatomy at the Medical College of Middlesex Hospital while operating a consultancy, specializing in the diagnosis and treatment of parasite-based diseases. In recognition of his voluminous work in systematic botany, comparative anatomy, and the natural history of worms, Cobbold was elected a fellow of the Royal Society in 1865. In 1873, he was appointed professor of botany at the Veterinary College of London, and later a special professorship in helminthology was created for him.[3]

For much of his career, Cobbold used publicity to create an audience for helminthology. During a lecture in Manchester, he insisted that no matter how distasteful worms might appear, they provided privileged access to the very workings of nature. From the study of "these little despised parasites," he stated, "there are teachings to be deduced which are in harmony with those derived from the more attractive sciences."[4] Health professionals were not spared Cobbold's zeal. Before the medical college at Middlesex Hospital, he deplored the ignorance of the medical profession about worms. "I have known the most erroneous statements have been made and published respecting their true nature, and have repeatedly received specimens from professional gentlemen, by post, for determination. Serious errors of practice have occasionally arisen from this source."[5]

Cobbold's use of the press as a rhetorical medium was not confined to creating a constituency for his specialty. It was no less critical in the creation of knowledge about worms. The press enabled Cobbold to transcend space to shape the narrative of discovery about parasites in the world without ever leaving London. In fact, Cobbold began documenting his encounter with the *filaria* worm while studying the eggs of the *Bilharzia haematobia* (*Schistosoma haemtobium*) worm in 1870. This trematode was a novelty for helminthologists when Theodore Bilharzia discovered it in 1851 in Cairo.[6] Bilharzia described the adult and the egg and connected their presence to a clinical disorder characterized by the discharge of blood into urine. Three years later, John Harley, a British doctor in Cape Colony, connected a similar disorder in South Africa to the presence of eggs that resembled Bilharzia's worm.[7]

Six years after Bilharzia's discovery, Cobbold proposed a revised nomenclature for the trematode: *Bilharzia haematobia*. Based on its general similarity to a large category of fluke worms, Bilharzia had designated his worm *Distoma haematobia*. But Cobbold and other helminthologists were dissatisfied with the general genus designation *Distomes*, particularly when new subspecies had been classified after its discovery. He recalled, "It was quite clear that its structural characters departed too strongly from those presented by the ordinary fluke-type to permit of its being zoologically associated with the Distomes properly so-called; consequently, various helminthologists proposed new and more appropriate names. . . . The choice of several systematists and others fell upon my title, which had the additional advantage of handling down the true discoverer's name to posterity." [8]

Later, the treatment of a girl for haematuria (or blood in the urine) from Natal province in 1870 enabled Cobbold to further shape the scientific narrative of the *Bilharzia* worm. In 1864, Harley had proposed a new subspecies of trematode (*Distoma capensis*) based on the appearance of a terminal spine on eggs instead of the lateral spine that Bilharzia had described. Cobbold, erroneously in retrospect, objected to the designation of a subspecies. The terminal spine, in Cobbold's opinion, was not a natural characteristic but an abnormality. In any case, Harley had failed to elaborate the complete life cycle of the parasite, that is, to identify the adult worm of the disputed egg and follow its development to maturity.[9]

It was while collecting *Bilharzia* eggs from his Natal case that Cobbold encountered several unknown immature forms. In an appendix to a paper on the *Bilharzia* worm, read before the Metropolitan Counties Branch of the British Medical Association in May 1872, Cobbold reported that "on five separate occasions, I obtained from the patient one or more specimens of the eggs or embryos of minute nematode." Without the parent worm, Cobbold was unable to identify these forms, but hoped that "future discoveries might enable us to identify this species of nematode to which these ova are referable." [10]

These ova attracted Cobbold's attention because of the possibility of placing a new urinary parasite on record. For Cobbold, worms that were responsible for diseases in humans or domesticated animals were highly effective vehicles for promoting the utility of helminthology to a broad range of potential constituencies, from medical practitioners, veterinarians, breeders, and farmers to the British public generally. Though he was reluctant to comment on the origins of the immature worms, Cobbold nevertheless attempted to bolster the possibility of a new discovery by analogy. Drawing on his encyclopedic knowledge of the literature on worms, in 1870 he yoked his unnamed finds to those of Dr. J. H. Salisbury of the United States. Salisbury, in 1868, had detected immature worms in three cases: once in the bladder and twice in the urine. Cobbold admitted there were differences between the two finds. Salisbury did not encounter his forms in haematuria cases, nor did Cobbold accept the provisional designation of Salisbury's worm—*Trichina cystica*—without the detection of the adult worm.[11]

In spite of these differences and in spite of the absence of the adult representative, Cobbold remained convinced that the immature forms that he obtained from his Natal patient "were identical with those of Dr. Salisbury, and referable to one and the same species of parasite." The fact that his case also hosted unrelated adult worms apparently lent credibility to the detection of a possibly new parasite. "It is not a little remarkable that the parents of my patient should have averred that she passed three small vermiform entozoa by the urethra; corresponding, judging from their verbal statements, very closely with the ordinary appearances of Filaria piscium. It is likewise worthy of note, that this patient had also played 'host' to about a dozen large lumbrici [or roundworms, known to infest the intestines]." [12]

Clearly, more was at stake than simply placing on record a potentially new urinary parasite. Why else would Cobbold go to such lengths to document the discovery of an unidentified worm retroactively? In referring to his 1870 detection in 1872, Cobbold was more than likely attempting to harness his find to the discovery of immature embryos in the urine and blood of a chylous case by Timothy Lewis in India. Cobbold could not ignore Lewis's discovery: The leading medical journals had devoted extensive coverage to the subject since 1870. Yet metropolitan attention was initially arrested not by the potential power of the parasite to illuminate disease per se but by Lewis's participation in the investigation into the cause of cholera under the sanitary commissioner with the government of India.

Spurred on by a cholera epidemic in 1867, this commission reflected the contentious politics of public health in India. As Mark Harrison has argued, the struggle over cholera control policy had major implications for the nature of British rule in India. Facing deficits and reluctant to provoke local unrest after the Indian Mutiny in 1857, the government of India, as a rule, adopted a policy of limited intervention. Government sanitary experts validated this policy largely by emphasizing that cholera was a localized disease. However, for advocates of the waterborne theory and quarantine, this policy, as well as its theoretical underpinnings, needlessly subordinated health to the fiscal and political imperatives of rule. [13]

The cholera commission was formed partly to justify official cholera policy by identifying a localized cause. To this end, the government of India and the British army agreed to select the best students from Netley to study the fungoid theory of Dr. Hallier of Jena and the subsoil theory of Max von Pettenkofer of Munich for six months. Based on their examination performances at Netley, Lewis and D. D. Cunningham were selected to represent the British army and the Indian Medical Service, respectively. [14] As Lewis and Cunningham proceeded to India in January 1869, an expectant audience in Britain and in India awaited the results of their investigations.

Not surprisingly, the publication of Lewis's report created a minor sensation in the metropolitan press. Although he did confirm the presence of Hallier's cysts and spores and micrococci in the stools and urine of cholera cases, experimentation proved these supposed pathogens to be harmless. Of Lewis's report, the *British Medical Journal* declared, "It is a document of permanent scientific interest, creditable to the author and to the service to which he belongs; and we commend it to the attention of all pathologists."[15] A month later, the *Lancet* added, "We cannot leave Dr. Lewis's report without expressing our conviction that the Indian Government have seldom done a wiser thing than in authorising the employment of himself and Dr. D. D. Cunningham in this most important inquiry."[16]

It was against this background that the *British Medical Journal* published a follow-up on Lewis's report that referred to the detection of ova in the urine in chylous cases. "In the valuable report on the microscopic objects found in cholera evacuations, to which we referred last week, Mr. T. R. Lewis gives an account of an observation of great interest made on a case of 'chylous urine.'" Lewis offered not definitive statements but qualified suggestions about the pathological significance and the zoological identity of the embryos:

Perhaps this fact may help throw some light on a very obscure disease, of which little is known beyond the symptoms, although frequently met with in some parts of the world; and indeed, may perhaps account for its localisation to such places as the West Coast of Africa, where, I am told, it is by no means a rare malady. As the mature worm still retains a hold on its victim, being perhaps safely lodged in the kidney—and I have not seen an embryo of this kind before, nor yet a drawing—I must leave to a more experienced helmintologist to decide to what species of nematode it belongs.[17]

Nearly a year and a half later, the press carried news of an even more startling find. In August 1872, Lewis informed the *Lancet* that he had detected embryos that survived in the bloodstream without being harmed or even debilitating the host. He also forwarded an embryo specimen to the *Lancet*. Moving quickly to confirm Lewis's find, the journal consulted George Busk, a leading authority on parasites and a surgeon on the hospital ship *Dreadnought*. Busk identified the embryos as "some kind of Filaria." Rather than waiting for identification of the adult worm, the *Lancet* gave a name to the new species: "It may not be inappropriate to christen the new entozoon 'Filaria sanguinis hominis.'"[18]

In the months that followed, the newly designated *filaria* worm received more exposure in the medical press. The *Lancet* published two further articles. One, in December, summarized the conclusions of Lewis's report on the haematozoa to the sanitary commissioner; a second, in January 1873, provided woodcuts and descriptions of the embryos.[19] In February, the *British Medical Journal* followed with a lead article in which it credited Lewis with discovering the first known human parasite adapted to live part of its life in the human bloodstream. "According to Mr. T. R. Lewis, to whom the honour of this discovery belongs, it appears that in certain individuals nematoids are 'persistently so ubiquitous as to be obtained day after day in numbers, by simply pricking any portion of the body, even to the tips of the fingers and toes and of both feet.' "[20]

Unlike the *Lancet*, the *British Medical Journal* pointed to gaps in the life cycle of the worm that needed to be filled before a definitive statement could be made regarding the relationship of the worm to chylous disease. These included the detection of the adult worm, the length of the embryos's stay in the blood, and the elaboration of the extracorporeal stage. Nevertheless, the lead article concluded on an encouraging note: "Mr Lewis's observations are of great value, and they clearly show, as he says, 'the importance of a careful microscopical examination of the blood of persons suffering from obscure diseases, in tropical countries especially.' They open up, in fact, a new and most important field of inquiry, which we hope will now be entered upon by many other observers."[21]

The publicity surrounding the *filaria* worm undoubtedly generated a considerable measure of pride among imperial doctors in India who had long resented their subordinate status in the British army and in the Indian Medical Services. Throughout the second half of the century, the medical profession at home and in India tried to browbeat the imperial state into improving the social conditions of doctors, that is, increasing their remuneration, addressing the backlog of promotion applications, securing for them rank equivalency, and greater authority over medical matters and public health. Editorials and letters asserted that the conditions of service discouraged better doctors, that is, graduates of English medical schools, from state service and thereby compromised the quality of health care in India. While effective in mobilizing professional opinion, this reform rhetoric perversely implied that imperial doctors were less competent than their colleagues in Britain, since a disproportionate number of them had graduated from Scottish and Irish medical schools.[22]

Lewis, a graduate of Aberdeen University, served as a model of what imperial doctors could do when given the resources and the opportunity. Anglo-Indian doctors were predictably sensitive to any perceived or manifest attempt to diminish or preempt the credit to Lewis for such an important discovery. This was particularly true of D. D. Cunningham, a member of the Indian Medical Service, who worked with Lewis while attached to the sanitary commissioner for the government of India. They collaborated chiefly on cholera, but Lewis turned to Cunningham for confirmation when he encountered embryos in the urine in 1870 and in the blood in 1872.[23]

In a strongly worded letter to the *Lancet* in June 1873, Cunningham protested against the association of Cobbold's finds with Lewis's. The cause of Cunningham's broadside was a study on the species identity of a canine *filaria* worm by Francis Welch, who served as an assistant professor at the Army Medical School, Netley. Lewis had encouraged just such a comparative study of a specimen at the pathological museum at Netley in order to shed further light on the natural history of a roundworm he had detected in 1870. But in a separate and supplementary section of Welch's report, he alluded to recent finds of nematoid ova and embryos in elephantiasis and other cases by Lewis and Cobbold among others. This was too close for comfort: Cunningham went out of his way to distinguish Lewis's discovery from Cobbold's. "Now Dr. Salisbury never discovered ova in chylous urine; (2) there is every evidence the ova and embryos in both Dr. Salisbury's and Dr. Cobbold's cases were mere accidents, and not true urinary parasites at all; and (3) even had they been so it is incorrect to state that Dr. Lewis's discovery was subsequent to [that of] Dr. Cobbold."[24]

Cunningham pointed out the discrepancy between the clinical condition of Salisbury's case and that of Lewis's. "It is evident that the only phenomenon in the case in any way resembling the phenomena of chyluria was *a milkiness due to a granular cystine*, a material hitherto not observed in connexion with chyluria" (emphasis in original). In a pointed rebuke to Cobbold, Cunningham noted that "it is somewhat astounding to find Dr. Cobbold, who 'unearthed' Salisbury's paper, confounding cystinuria with chyluria." He added, "If every case in which the urine contains whitish suspended matter is to be styled one of chyluria, the disease will be found to be much more widely diffused than it has hitherto been considered to be."

To Cunningham, the clinical conditions associated with the finds of Salisbury and Cobbold suggested the common intestinal parasite *Oxyuris vermicularis* rather than the *filaria* worm. Cobbold apparently overlooked the common gender of the cases and their special relationship to intestinal parasites. "Now it has long been on record that it is in females that intestinal entozoa, their ova and embryos, are liable to obtain accidental entrance into the urine, the anatomical relations of the digestive and urinary apparatus being such as to facilitate the wandering of entozoa from the former into the latter." Clinical signs, such as the "dribbling" of fluid or the "passing of a small vermiform entozoa" from the urethra, should have alerted Cobbold to the possible presence of an intestinal parasite. "Judging by verbal statements between parasites so minute as Filaria piscium and Oxyuris vermicularis is ticklish work," Cunningham sarcastically observed, "and it is amusing to find Dr. Cobbold, in his haste to discover some new and startling relationship between his ova and embryos, neglecting to take the common parasite into consideration."[25]

From Cunningham's point of view, Cobbold exaggerated the significance of the ova and embryos he encountered in the urine of his Natal case. "The accidental occurrence of the ova or embryos of entozoa in urine is a fact regarding which observations have long been on record, and it is incredible that any dispute should arise at the present day regarding the right of priority of discovery of it." This was hardly the basis for a discovery. "Almost as well might a discussion be raised regarding the right of priority in the discovery of cotton fibres in urine." Even in the unlikely event that Cobbold had indeed observed immature *filariae*, Lewis had been first to publish. "Dr. Lewis's Report, in its original form, is dated April 1870, and the paragraphs relating to the filaria were reprinted in full in the British Medical Journal of the 19th November, 1870, and referred to in other journals at an earlier date."[26]

For his part, Welch resented the insinuation that he worked in league with Cobbold. Defensively, he explained that "the paragraph, as its opening words express, is a mere noting of those occasions on which the existence of larvae and ova of *nematoid worms in human fluids* has been demonstrated, and terminating with the mention of the *filariae*—two distinct subjects." Evidently, Cunningham's overheated imagination saw mischief where none could possibly exist.

Whether the nematoid ova of Salisbury and Cobbold were true urinary parasites is a matter to be determined by those who have made the subject a study, yet until these ova are found to be the egg stage of Lewis's filaria (a point asserted by no one, and negativated by contrast of the worms), I am at a loss to understand how the honour of the discovery of the filariae, and the elucidation of their pathological bearings can suffer tarnish by the detection in the urine, whether before or after, of ova and larvae of an entirely different worm, with no certain pathological concomitants![27]

Cunningham's fears proved prophetic. Less than a year and a half later, the unknown immature forms that Cobbold detected in 1870 ceased being the progeny of a possibly new urinary parasite. Instead, they became identical to the *microfilariae* detected by Lewis. Ironically, Lewis furnished Cobbold with just the pretext he needed to assert a generic identity between the immature forms. Perhaps as a gesture to mend fences after Cunningham's broadside,

Lewis forwarded to Cobbold a copy of his study on canine *filariae* in late 1874.[28] As we will see, this gesture backfired.

In a letter to the *Lancet*, ostensibly about Lewis's latest report, Cobbold informed readers that the recently discovered human *filaria* was not so original after all. "It will be within the recollection of most persons that Sir William Jenner exhibited to the Pathological Society some of the haematozoa originally discovered by Dr. Lewis in human blood." Cobbold did not stop here. Unlike Welch, who grouped nematodes found in body fluids to illuminate the similarities between allied species of human and canine *filariae*, Cobbold unilaterally asserted a common identity between his parasites and those of Lewis. In particular, he pressed into service the find of Sonsino Prospero, an Italian physician in Egypt. Although Prospero reported stumbling onto nematoid worms while searching for *Bilharzia*, he did not relate them to the *microfilaria*. "It is only fair," Cobbold noted, "to mention that Dr. Prospero Sonsino, of Cairo . . . has also found nematodes in the human blood, and since they were associated (as in my own case) with the presence of *Bilharzia haematobia*, there can be little doubt that they refer to the same parasite as that discovered by Lewis." After this leap, Cobbold made another: "In short, the human nematode worms from the blood and urine found by Salisbury and myself are without doubt referable to the so-called *Filaria sanguinis hominis*." [29]

Cobbold reiterated his assertion a year later, in 1876, when announcing that Joseph Bancroft, Sr., of Brisbane, Queensland, Australia, had discovered immature worms. By way of William Roberts, a renal specialist based in Manchester, Cobbold received several tubes containing blood from a chylous case under Bancroft's care. Cobbold reported: "I detected about twenty filariae, three of which I sketched *in situ*, in order to compare them with the figures of Lewis, and also with others that I procured from my *Bilharzia* patient in the year 1870. There cannot, I think, be much doubt as to the identity of all of these sexually immature nematoids." The presence of a "solitary and empty shell," which measured the same size as the ova he had observed in his Natal case, removed any doubt from his mind. Even though Sonsino doubted the relationship between his and Lewis's finds, Cobbold persisted in bundling them together. "On comparing my drawings with those given by Dr. Sonsino, in his 'Researches concerning *Bilharzia haematobia* in relation to the endemic *haematuria* in Egypt, with a notice respecting a nematoid in the human blood . . .' I find that they might almost be made to do duty the one for the other." [30]

Until the fall of 1877, Lewis remained unmoved by Cobbold's selective record of discovery. Neither the Anglo-Indian nor the metropolitan medical press acknowledged the authenticity of Cobbold's claims. But Lewis did clash with Cobbold in print over the question of priority of discovery of the adult representative of the *filaria*. In April 1877, Bancroft wrote to Cobbold that he had detected the long-sought parental worm in five cases. He promised to forward a full description, as well as specimens, as soon as he found "a trustworthy messenger."[31] Rather than waiting for Bancroft's parcel, Cobbold went public. In his letter to the *Lancet* announcing the discovery, Cobbold immodestly described his own participation in the detection of the adult worm. Shortly after Cobbold detected embryos in blood specimens forwarded by Bancroft in April 1876, Cobbold urged Bancroft to search for the adult. This advice, contained in an article in the *Veterinarian*, "induced [Bancroft] to continue his investigations. These further researches have resulted in the record of novel facts, which, in response to his courtesy, I now make public."[32] Flushed with the seemingly unproblematic discovery of the adult worm, Cobbold proposed to designate the adult worm, in recognition of his collaborator, *Filaria Bancrofti*.[33]

Doubts about the identity of Bancroft's worm surfaced soon after Cobbold's announcement. Less than two months later, Lewis detected two adult worms in a blood clot from a scrotal case. Lewis, unlike Cobbold, provided a detailed anatomical description. Strategically, this difference was important because, through comparative anatomy, Lewis was now able to determine whether Cobbold's find in his Natal patient could be construed as the offspring of an adult representative of the *filaria* worm. Cobbold had described the tube that enveloped the immature ova as a "shell," which implied an oviparous parent. But uterine tubules filled with "ova in various stages of development" indicated a viviparous parent. Further, the "shell" that Cobbold claimed to see was in fact the distinctive sac of the immature worm while in the bloodstream. "The ova do not possess any distinctly marked 'shell'; from the smallest to the largest nothing but a delicate pellicle can be distinguished as enveloping the embryo in all its stages."[34]

From Lewis's perspective, there was no reason to give the adult worm a special name. Whether Bancroft's worm was identical to Lewis's remained an open question. Cobbold's announcement did not allow for a systematic comparison of the worms. In any case, a genus nomenclature had already been adopted. "I have retained for the mature parasite the name originally applied to the embryo—applied obviously on the supposition that sooner or later the parent would be forthcoming." Lewis reminded Cobbold that other naturalists in Europe found little amiss with the designation. "As it has, moreover, already been adopted by Leuckart in his recently complete standard work 'On Parasites,' and by other continental authorities, a new name, if not necessary on anatomical grounds, would only lead to confusion."[35]

Known for "the courage of his opinions," Cobbold did not back down.[36] After reviewing the two worms, he was all the more convinced that they were identical. In spite of the meager details in his announcement, Cobbold defended his nomenclature in the name of zoological custom. "As regards the nomenclature, I have associated Dr. Bancroft's name with the sexually mature worm as being in harmony with the binomial method and little calculated to mislead." He added that it "fixed both the source and date of discovery (Brisbane, Dec. 21st, 1876)." Cobbold claimed that this "concession" to Bancroft "detracts nothing from the higher merits of Lewis, who was the first to name the immature worm, *Filaria sanguinis hominis*." [34]

In the same breath, Cobbold diminished Lewis's claim to priority in discovering the immature embryo by asserting, again, a generic identity between the finds of Lewis and of Salisbury. "Should my determination of the genetic relationship of [Lewis's] embryos with *Filaria Bancrofti* be subsequently verified, it would obviously be absurd to call the adult worm *Trichina cystica*; yet Salisbury gave this name to the urinary parasite." In an appendix to his article, Cobbold insisted that "all of the various larval forms severally described by Salisbury, Lewis, Sonsino, Wucherer, Crevaux and Corre, Silva-Lima, Bancroft and myself, are referable to one and the same species." Having reiterated his version of priority, Cobbold disingenuously offered no personal objection to the adoption of "Lewis's trinomial name . . . in place of *Filaria Bancrofti*." He, nevertheless, continued using the latter term, which remains a part of the systematic nomenclature of the worm to this day.[38]

Was Manson unaware of this running dispute? At first sight, it would appear so. He makes no reference to it in his reading notebook. Yet it is unlikely that Manson remained totally unaware of the conflict between Lewis and Cobbold. Before, during, and after Manson's furlough, the metropolitan press carried the thrust of Cobbold and the parry of Lewis as the life cycle of the *filaria* worm unfolded. If Manson did not know, it is hard to explain why he solicited the advice of the two principals regarding the discovery of the mosquito as intermediary host.

The Rhetoric and Spectacle of the Mosquito as Intermediary Host

On 27 November 1877, Manson solicited Cobbold's advice: "I live in an out-of-the-world place, away from libraries, and out of the run of what is going on, so that I do not know very well the value of my work, or if it has been done before, or better." [39] Manson was not an unknown quantity to Cobbold. Months earlier,

Manson had sent a reprint of his study on canine *filariae* to T. B. Curling, a specialist in the disease in the suprapubic region. Curling, in turn, had forwarded the report to Cobbold in October. On 4 January, Manson's parcel arrived. Its contents included his epidemiological study of human *filaria* in Amoy, as well as slide preparations of embryos and larvae from sectioned mosquitoes that had fed on Hin-Lo's blood. Cobbold examined the contents, then announced the discovery of the intermediary host in the *Lancet* a week later.[40]

Cobbold made little effort to experimentally verify Manson's discovery before going public. Even if he had wanted to, there were practical difficulties, namely, the paucity of clinical cases infected with *microfilariae* and of suitable mosquitoes. Given the rapidly unfolding life history of the worm, Cobbold was eager to associate himself with another critical moment in the narrative of discovery. He wrote that Joseph Bancroft, in April 1877, had "wondered if mosquitoes could suck up the haematozoa and convey them to water," but added, "Whether or not this conception of the possible host-parasite relationship, as between man and mosquito, primarily originated with Bancroft or some other observer I cannot stop to inquire, but certain it is that what Bancroft surmised Dr. Manson has demonstrated to be a fact." [41]

For Cobbold, being first was its own reward. But the use of the press to establish priority politicized the process of discovery. Cobbold had claimed the priority of discovery for different stages of the worm's life cycle. He unilaterally revised the sequence of discovery of the *microfilariae* and announced the discovery of the adult representative based on a manifestly incomplete record. Although this public style of science was effective in staking out priority, it problematized verification. Raising doubts about a new "fact" amounted to questioning the credibility of its endorser as well as its discoverer. Paradoxically, when Manson solicited the advice of Cobbold and Lewis, he created the conditions for a possible confrontation between the two. Unlike Cobbold, Lewis, in India, was in a position to confirm or deny Manson's sequence of *filaria* development in the mosquito.

Initially, Lewis was guarded in his reply to Manson. He congratulated Manson on his "interesting observation regarding the embryonic nematode in the mosquito," but stopped short of endorsing the mosquito as intermediary host. Without any basis for evaluating Manson's slide preparations, Lewis was reluctant to affirm that the forms were referable to the *F. sanguinis hominis*. "Whether they are actually identical or not it would, perhaps, hardly be safe to assert positively without further experience, but given slides with specimens of each kind I should be very sorry to be asked to decide which had been derived from the mosquito and which from man." Lewis also warned Manson of the possibility of conflating embryos and larvae of *filaria* with others that call the mosquito home. "With regard to the larger parasites to which you refer, you will doubtless be aware that the mosquito, like nearly all insects, occasionally harbours different kinds of parasites. It will, of course, occur to you that due consideration of this circumstance is of prime importance in drawing any inference as to the generic connexion between the various parasites observed." [42]

Soon after receiving Manson's letter, Lewis attempted to verify experimentally *filaria* development in the mosquito. Even though Lewis duplicated Manson's biting experiment, he could not verify the advanced embryo or larva stage that Manson claimed to see, nor could he confirm that water was the medium of development outside the mosquito. Lewis failed not because he was inexperienced but, rather, because he was a more exacting experimenter. Like Manson, he assumed that the mosquito reproduced and died within a week after its single blood meal. The practical result of this assumption terminated larval development by starving the mosquito to death. As a result, Lewis could observe only one-third of the optimal size of larvae in the mosquito. Nor was there any possibility of confirming, much less imagining, Manson's advanced water stage, since Lewis confined his weeklong search to the abdominal and thoracic cavities of his mosquitoes and therefore could not commingle larvae that were older than a week and/or were lodged in the salivary glands of the mosquito's proboscis. [43]

Lewis conducted two experiments, which he reported to the Asiatic Society of Bengal. The first produced little evidence of development in the mosquito. After three days, he noticed that the embryos in the stomach had "succumbed to the digestive action of the insect's stomach." By the fourth and fifth days, there was little or no evidence of haematozoalike forms. However, in a second experiment a week later, he examined the muscle tissues of a mosquito. In this experiment, which was published as an addendum to his report, Lewis found that some of the ingested embryos were digested by the stomach acids and "others actually perforate the walls of the insect's stomach, pass out, and then undergo developmental stages in the thoracic and abdominal tissues." [44] By the fourth day, Lewis had confirmed Manson's sausage stage in the thoracic cavity. "About the fourth day there will be seen short, thick bodies (very appropriately described by Dr. Manson as 'sausage-shaped'), almost perfectly still . . . with a faint mouth, and in some of them, a fainter line may be detected suggestive of a commencing intestinal canal; the escape of a few granules on slight pressure towards the other, usually thicker, suggests the existence of an anal aperture." [45]

During the remainder of the fourth day and the fifth day, however, Lewis

obtained results that materially differed from Manson's sequence of development. Although the larvae underwent extensive growth, they were consider-
ably smaller than Manson's measurements. More important, Lewis found that
his most advanced larvae possessed only a limited amount of physiological differentiation. "When examined in the unbroken condition it is only with difficulty that the alimentary canal can be distinguished beyond the junction of the
oesophagus with the intestine, but when carefully ruptured . . . the tube may be
distinguished. I have not been able to distinguish other differentiated viscus in
any of the specimens which have come under my observation, and, certainly,
nothing suggestive of differentiation of sex." [46]

By the fifth day, these immature worms were simply too fragile to lead an
independent existence anywhere, much less in water as Manson had speculated. Careful searches for larvae in the water where the mosquito deposited
her eggs and/or died proved fruitless. "Either no *filariae* were found in [the
mosquito's] body, or if present they were dead, and careful examination of the
water invariably yielded negative results in my hand." Although he conceded
that his procedures may have doomed his results, he concluded, "I cannot as a
result of personal observation affirm that a sojourn in the body of the mosquito,
and subsequent transference to water, suffice to bring the *Filaria sanguinis
hominis* to maturity." [47]

Lewis's conclusion echoed throughout the metropolitan press. The *British
Medical Journal* wondered, "Is the Mosquito the Intermediary Host?" [48] The
Medical Times and Gazette cautioned readers that "recent observations
would seem to disprove or to render very doubtful the theory that the mosquito acts . . . as the particular intermediate host of the *Filaria sanguinis
hominis*." [49] A review in *Nature* of Lewis's monograph on microscopic organisms concluded that "the hypothesis of Manson concerning the part played by
mosquitoes as intermediate hosts (within which some of the embryos swallowed may undergo development, and from the bodies of which parent forms,
capable of infecting man, find their way into drinking water) seems, from the
careful observations made by Lewis, to be rendered more than doubtful." [50]

Cobbold was now in a difficult position. He could not experimentally verify
Manson's report, nor was he prepared to retract his statement. Instead, he went
on the offensive by selectively interpreting Lewis's experiment. Since Lewis
had verified Manson's "sausage" stage, his concerns about the immaturity of
the larvae needlessly obscured the obvious. "With the caution of a true savant,
Dr. Lewis gives only qualified assent to Manson's discovery, observing that 'it
cannot be said that even these later observations (of his own) are sufficiently
conclusive to warrant a positive statement being made.' Dr. Lewis says that

'no trace of reproductive organs' is distinguishable in the embryos from the mosquito. Had my Linnean paper appeared I think he would have come to a different conclusion." [51]

But neither in Cobbold's paper nor in Manson's report are the reproductive organs described.[52] Manson himself was unsure whether the opening adjacent to the caudal opening was "the head or tail, and whether the vessel opening near it the alimentary canal or vagina." [53] Although he speculated in a later paper in 1884 that a vacuole behind the mouth and line of cells suggested respectively a vagina and the latter organs of reproduction, Manson admitted that these suggestions were based only on a "solitary observation" to which he attached "no great weight." [54]

Like Cobbold, Manson buttressed his discovery rhetorically. In a letter to the *Medical Times and Gazette*, he recast Lewis's observations to prove that the mosquito was the intermediary host. Just as Lewis had earlier warned Manson of the possibility of confusing different parasites in the mosquito, Manson claimed that Lewis had conflated canine *filariae* with human *filariae* in his first experiment. "Now, as he took no particular steps to insure his mosquitoes feeding on human blood, it is more than probable that the insects he first examined, and which he himself says were captured at random, contained dog-haematozoa, and not *Filaria sanguinis hominis*." For Manson, the fact that Lewis later succeeded in verifying some development in the second experiment simply confirmed the role of the mosquito. "The inference from this is obvious. Dr. Lewis observed in his mosquitoes, in the first instance the digestion of canine haematozoa, and in the second instance the development of human haematozoa. I fail to see how these observations tend to disprove or render very doubtful the theory that the mosquito acts as the intermediary host of *Filaria sanguinis hominis*." Nor did Manson regard the immaturity of larvae or the limited number of advanced forms as particularly problematic. "That a few do advance is sufficient to prove the mosquito a promoter of developmental changes, and if we find that these changes are carried sufficiently far to make independent existence possible just at the time of death of the mosquito renders an independent existence necessary, the inference that the mosquito is the proper intermediary host cannot be avoided." Manson was confident that he would be vindicated shortly. "This has been found, and I have little doubt that many observers in India and elsewhere have by this time amply confirmed my statements." [55]

In the meantime, Manson offered additional circumstantial evidence that the mosquito was the intermediary host. During his epidemiological study on *filariae* in Amoy in mid-1877, Manson commented on an anomaly regarding the behavior of *microfilariae* in the bloodstream. In eighty-nine cases, he noticed that *filariae* embryos were temporarily absent in thirty-four and present in fifty-five. At this time, Manson speculated that this curious phenomenon resulted from the disruption of the reproductive behavior of the parent worm caused by death or by the formation of a cyst.[56]

A year and a half later, Manson returned to the behavior of the *microfilariae*. He trained two hospital assistants to examine the blood and record the number of embryos observed as part of their regular duties, one in the evening and the other during the day. Almost immediately, Manson noticed a distinction between the daytime and nighttime observations. "On some days there appeared to be great abundance of *filariae*, on other days none, or very few. I noticed that when they were abundant, the examination was made on busy days, when there was much work to be done in the hospital, and extra work of this sort had to be got through in the evening; and that when they were absent, the examination was made during the day."[57]

Doubting that this distinction was more than an accident, Manson began systematically examining the blood of infected patients every four hours. The results were startling. Based on the blood examinations, Manson inferred that "*filaria* embryos invariably begin to appear in the circulation at sunset, their numbers gradually increase till about midnight, during the early morning they become fewer by degrees, and by 9 or 10 o'clock in the forenoon it is very rare to find one in the blood." Manson drew a direct inference from this phenomenon to the customary feeding habits of the female mosquito. "For the meaning of it I think we have not far to look. The nocturnal habits of the *[F]ilaria sanguinis hominis* are adapted to the nocturnal habits of the mosquito, its intermediary host, and is only another of the many wonderful instances of adaptation so constantly met with in nature."[58]

Since Cobbold had responded so warmly to his description of *filaria* development in the mosquito, it should hardly come as a surprise that Manson solicited his advice rather than Lewis's. Manson wrote in June 1879, "If you find these notes of value in any way, I should be pleased you should make what use you like of them." Cobbold did: He promptly communicated them to the Queckett Microscopical Society, where he had presided since 1879.[59]

Cobbold presented Manson's latest report as part of a research overview of the life history of the *filaria*. Predictably, it favored Cobbold's version of priority. He included himself and Salisbury among the circle of discoverers of the *microfilaria* and noted his participation in the detection of the adult representative. "Guided by certain indications which I pointed out to him, Dr. Joseph Bancroft, as he has acknowledged, sought for and discovered the adult worm on the 21st of December, 1876. He wished me to publish his very short notice of the worm, because, as he said, 'I had set him on the track of the investigation.' " Even though Cobbold conceded that Lewis's description of the adult worm had been in print earlier, he perversely offered to give up his genus nomenclature, that is, *Filaria Bancrofti*, but "with the distinct understanding, however, that such a step shall not deprive my Brisbane correspondent of the honor of priority in this matter." [60]

When presenting Manson's report on the periodicity of *microfilariae*, Cobbold framed it as a further elaboration of Manson's discovery of the mosquito as intermediary host. Even though Lewis publicly doubted Manson's discovery, Cobbold implied the opposite. "I may add that since the issue of my treatise, Dr. Lewis has published a beautifully illustrated memoir in which he not only verifies a great deal of what Dr. Manson has already observed, but adds a multitude of interesting details." For Cobbold, periodicity represented another novel fact, one that explained why previous investigators had had difficulty detecting the *microfilariae* in the human bloodstream and fortified the hypothesis of its adaptive relationship with the mosquito. "Dr. Manson explains how it happens that human blood does not contain *Filariae* during the afternoon. He gives a tabular record of the results of the daily examination of the blood at different hours. He shows how the embryos, with almost military punctuality, march to their nocturnal quarters. Proofs of this extraordinary behavior are supplied by repeated observations." [61]

Filarial periodicity by itself did not necessarily reverse opinion about the role of the mosquito as intermediary host. To be sure, the metropolitan press, including the *Queckett Journal*, the *Lancet*, and the *Transactions of the Pathological Society*, carried news about Manson's latest discovery.[62] But the public demonstration of periodicity in London by Stephen Mackenzie on 18 October 1882 proved decisive. The presentation of a European infected with living *microfilariae* before a packed audience at the Pathological Society afforded an opportunity to constitute the life history of the worm. Here was a case in which seeing was believing.

Mackenzie was not a specialist in tropical diseases per se, but a skin specialist at London Hospital. He, like other metropolitan specialists, was particularly interested in *filariasis*.[63] Besides following the coverage of Lewis's discovery in the medical press, Mackenzie was present in May 1881 at the Pathological Society meeting where George Thin communicated a paper by Manson.[64] In this paper, which was supplemented by the first adult worm specimen lodged in a lymphatic vessel, Manson discussed the evening behavior of *microfilariae*.[65] Mackenzie's own encounter with living specimens of *filaria* occurred in the summer, when Dr. Ralf, a colleague at London Hospital, admitted an enlisted soldier from India suffering from chyluria. Aware of Mackenzie's interest in the disease, Ralf transferred the case to him.[66]

This case provided Mackenzie with a rare opportunity to study the condition as well as to search for *microfilariae*. Once Mackenzie had detected *microfilariae*, in early August, he used his clinical case as an opportunity to confirm its periodicity. From August until January, Mackenzie and his assistant, Mr. Coates, systematically observed the blood of the patient every three hours. Coates, who performed much of the evening labor, noticed an unvarying pattern in the numbers of *microfilariae*: They increased from 9 P.M. to 3 A.M. and declined to nothing from 3 A.M. to 6 P.M. To underscore the behavior of the immature worms, they reversed the eating and sleeping time of the patient from evening to day. This change had the effect of inverting the usual behavior of *microfilariae* in the blood: more were present in the day than in the evening.[67]

Mackenzie discussed his finding at the Pathological Society on 18 October.[68] Although the exhibition of a clinical case to illustrate a diagnosis or procedure was a routine practice at the Society, it is likely that Mackenzie's case captured the imagination of the audience. The Anglo-Indian patient appeared "to be in good health," but his body teemed with *microfilariae*. By one calculation, some "36,000,000 to 40,000,000" coursed through his bloodstream during the evening.[69] Slide preparations and microphotographs of the patient's blood permitted observation of the worm in its human host. This visual representation of the worm not only supplemented Mackenzie's presentation but also enhanced the truth value of its life history. "The *filariae* as shown were identical with those which he saw in Amoy with Dr. Manson," testified Walter Pye.[70] "The members of the Pathological Society," a report in the *Lancet* raved, "enjoyed the rare opportunity (in this country) of seeing the *Filaria sanguinis hominis* in the living state from a patient in the London Hospital suffering from haemato-chyluria, under the care of Dr. Stephen MacKenzie."[71]

An infected European, seemingly in good health, and living *filariae* specimens were not the only visual novelties that evening. Mackenzie, with Cobbold's permission, exhibited sectioned mosquitoes that contained embryo and larvae-stage *filariae*. The geographical diversity of these specimens, which had originated in Australia, China, and India, visually underscored an adaptive, biological relationship between mosquito, worm, and human.[72] Acting as the evening's docent, Cobbold authenticated what the audience observed. Seeking dramatic effect, he portrayed the discovery of the mosquito and filarial periodicity as the fourth and fifth "epochs" in the elaboration of the life history of the worm.

The first was the urinary *filariae* in 1866. Then in 1872 Lewis found these parasites in chylurious patients and others in various tissues of the body. The next epoch was Bancroft's discovery, in Australia, of the sexually mature worm, three and a half inches long, in a lymphatic abscess in the arm; six months after Lewis in India, and Manson in China and in Brazil. The fourth epoch was Manson's discovery of the intermediary host, the mosquito. The fifth and last epoch is the discovery of filarial periodicity by Manson.[73]

Direct observation in London validated the mosquito as host. Even Lewis's observations, which had earlier rendered Manson's discovery doubtful, were now invoked in Manson's support. "The mosquito feeding on the blood at night, when the *filariae* are generally alone to be found, becomes gorged with them. Their growth in the mosquito has been traced by Lewis and Manson, and it is presumed that they are only liberated from the body of their host by its death in the water to which it always finally resorts."[74]

Mackenzie's presentation represented an important turning point in the discovery of the intermediary host of the *Filaria* worm. At least in London, where it mattered, there was little doubt about the role of the mosquito. To be sure, Manson had been convinced all along of the validity of his discovery. But he now had even less reason to question his experimental and rhetorical practices. If anything, the conflicting observations of Lewis and other investigators became a source of irritation, rather than a point of departure for a critical evaluation of his underlying conviction.[75]

Lingering doubts among continental researchers about the mosquito as intermediary host induced Manson to undertake a second biting experiment in 1884.

Some eminent helminthologists in England accept my statements and endorse the inferences I have drawn—Cobbold for example. But in other quarters, so far from securing acceptance of my theory, the work of Lewis, on account of the hesitation and scientific caution with which he expresses himself, has had the effect of inducing a certain amount of scepticism. Leuckart is sceptical; and of course scepticism of so eminent an authority is of great weight in influencing opinion, especially in Germany. Some of our zoologists, also, I understand, share the views of Leuckart.

By repeating his experiment, Manson hoped to do a service to medicine and helminthology and "settle the matter."[76]

To this end, Manson significantly altered the rhetoric organization of his report. He not only provided illustrations but also forwarded slide preparations to "friends in England and elsewhere." These slides, he hoped, "should the frail structures they contain retain the appearances they had when they left my hands, cannot fail to satisfy the most cautious and scientific mind." Manson also enlisted the "testimony" of two "perfectly competent judges from Amoy, Drs. Macleish and McDougall," who viewed his experiments and preparations.[77] Moreover, Manson's language of experimental science changed as well. Unlike his first report, his second exuded expertise. It exhibited a consciousness of the artificiality of experimental observation, openly admitted speculation when discussing unknown objections and their functions, registered an increase in the level of detail, and engaged the reader in considering possible hazards to be avoided.

For all Manson's efforts to authenticate his findings, he did not bother to alter the basic design of the experiment. His mosquitoes were wild. Even though he insisted that he "took care that [their] only food was the blood of a filariated man," he attracted them in much the same way as he had in his first experiment in 1877.[78] Mosquitoes entered a specially built mosquito house in the evening and gorged themselves on the blood of a sleeping infected human subject. They were then trapped by closing the door; later, Manson's assistant collected and placed them in glass bottles, noting the time and date. Over the course of several weeks, Manson amassed hundreds, possibly thousands, of mosquitoes. While this collection method ensured that the mosquitoes fed on the one human subject, this did not mean that they had not ingested *filariae* during previous blood meals.

So too did Manson's representation of development remain largely unchanged. He did adopt Lewis's technique of dissecting the cavities of the mosquito from abdomen to thorax. Over the course of seven days, he observed embryos shedding their sheaths within an hour after ingestion, the formation of digestive and reproductive organs in larvae beginning on the third day, and the transformation of the fragile and inert sausage form to an animal capable of independent locomotion between the fourth and seventh days.

Manson continued to group his observations into stages of development, though he acknowledged that these were artificial. "The reader must bear in mind," he remarked in a footnote, "that this division of the metamorphosis is entirely artificial. No such thing exists in nature. What I describe as stages, in reality overlap each other; the graduations of development insensibly merge one into another."[79] As in the narrative of his first experiment, these stages, which he increased from three to six, glossed over the appearance of more than one generation of larvae in a single mosquito. In fact, Manson pointed to this anomaly in support of the transformation of embryos to advanced larvae: "Besides being able to trace the gradation of different ages, we often encounter specimens of the *Filaria*, at all stages of development from fig. 3 to fig. 14, in one and the same mosquito. Sometimes in an insect in which a *Filaria* like fig. 14 is found, many others, at all stages of development, from fig. 14 to fig. 24, may be encountered. And so with the latest stages: fig. 23 may be found in a slide in which fig. 33 is moving."[80]

Ironically, it was these experimental practices that prevented others from replicating Manson's sequence of development in the mosquito. Without laboratory-bred mosquitoes, following morphological change required a series of highly subjective judgments. While the mosquito hosted more than one parasite, sustained observation allowed for a measure of familiarity with the *microfilariae* and early larvae stages. But even Manson acknowledged that morphological changes were rapid and hard to follow. Further, systematic searches of the abdominal and thoracic cavities were of only limited usefulness. The death of the mosquito from starvation prevented the larvae from growing larger than a little more than one-third to one-half their optimal size. In sum, only Manson could see what he reported.

*   *   *

Even though no one verified Manson's sequence of development in entirety, the mosquito became a part of the established narrative of the worm's life history. Manson prevailed due to the explanatory power of experimental science and the centrality of the metropolitan medical press in constituting imperial knowledge. By facilitating the priority dispute between Cobbold and Lewis, the medical press had created an audience for the *filaria* worm and framed the reception of Manson's flawed discovery. The contrasting verdicts about the role of the mosquito reached by Lewis and Cobbold produced a showdown at the Pathological Society.

Here, Manson prevailed in spite of experimental science that questioned the role of the mosquito as intermediary host. Stephen Mackenzie's presentation of filarial periodicity provided an opportunity to reconstruct the life history of the *filaria* worm in London. The observation of living specimens, together with the exhibition of sectioned mosquitoes containing embryos and larvae, naturalized the human body and the mosquito as host and intermediary host, respectively. As the *Lancet* report of the meeting indicated, this spectacle displaced the doubts that Lewis had raised and vindicated Cobbold's original announcement on behalf of Manson.

Moreover, Cobbold used the pages of other metropolitan periodicals, as well as his own textbook on worms, to establish his version of scientific priority: He marginalized Lewis's criticism.[81] Outside of Britain, the circulation of Cobbold's narrative of discovery fortified the role of the mosquito as intermediary host. Dr. Bourel-Roncière's report on the *filaria* worm in the French armed services medical journal, *Archives de Medecine Navale*, made no reference to the inconsistencies in Manson's sequence of development.[82] Neither did Maurice Nielly, in his *Elements de Pathologie Exotique*.[83] Nor do they appear in the prize essay of American entomologist C. R. Arron on the destruction of the mosquito. In fact, Arron cited an account of Lewis's verification report to underscore the role of mosquitoes in transmitting human disease.[84] So did Charles-Louis-Alphonse Laveran, a French military surgeon in colonial Algeria. Laveran proposed that the mosquito might play a similar role in the development and transmission of his recently identified malaria parasite.[85]

The attention that Manson received must have been gratifying despite the defensive tone he adopted in his second Linnean report. The reception to the republication in book form of his articles on the pathology, epidemiology, and natural history of the *filaria* worm in 1883 was favorable. A review in the *British Medical Journal* observed, "The name of Dr. Manson is well known in medical and scientific circles in England and on the Continent of Europe. During a lengthened career in China, he has earned the reputation of being a keen investigator and accurate observer as well as a medical man of great practical attainment."[86] Of the investigators pursuing the *filaria*, a reviewer for the *Veterinarian* declared, "Foremost amongst the workers in this field stands the name of Dr. Manson. . . . Dr. Manson's labours have been continuous and incessant, and only those who have watched the development of the whole subject can adequately appreciate its importance in relation to medicine."[87]

This recognition came at a fortuitous time in his career. After nearly twenty years in practice in China, Manson decided to retire. Henrietta explained, "Health was one reason, as he was customarily getting attacks of gout and had headaches. He wanted rest and to be at home with his children."[88] Money certainly was not a factor. Before returning to Britain in 1889, he had spent three lucrative years in practice in Hong Kong, provided contract services for steamboat companies, and served on the colonial government medical board. Manson had prospered, generating £5,000 per year, a sum of money that only the very elite doctors of London could claim to earn. This sum, together with his previous earnings in silver from Amoy, would have permitted a very comfortable retirement.[89]

Manson's remaining years in Hong Kong were active quite apart from his thriving practice. He wanted to leave a legacy after spending nearly two decades in China. To this end, he became the chief organizer of the Alice Marble Medical College and the Hong Kong Medical Society, and he served as their dean and president, respectively.[90] These forays into institution building brought closure to Manson's long-term concerns, namely, the diffusion of Western medicine and the protection of the economic rewards of the profession. The medical college provided professional instruction to Chinese students without the obstacles of mission medicine while promoting westernization. The medical society served as a pressure group to protect the economic interest of the profession. It sought legal remedy for members from nonpaying patients and attempted to curb charitable medicine by urging the colonial government to appoint a salaried medical officer for the poor.[91]

Shortly after returning to Britain, Manson found he had to defer his plans to retire to Scotland. Concentrating his retirement capital in Chinese silver currency had been ill-advised because gold had supplanted silver as the most stable world currency by the 1880s. The value of silver became even more unstable just as Manson moved his family to Britain. Quite apart from the diminution of his standard of living, the prospects of his son and two daughters were now imperiled. No future could be stable based on the value of a declining investment. Manson had little choice but to prolong his career in medicine.

Manson could not launch a second career just anywhere. There were a number of considerations. Gout and his advancing age ruled out a return to China. Prospects in Scotland were not particularly auspicious, either. Manson did receive an honorary doctorate of laws from Aberdeen University for his contributions to tropical medicine. Still, this was hardly an appropriate specialty for the relatively small medical market of Aberdeen. Manson had little alternative but to pursue a practice in London. To this end, in 1890 he secured a qualification from the Royal College of Physicians.[92]

London proved to be an ideal place for Manson. London represented the administrative-political center of the British empire and the center of imperial medicine. As Britain's territorial reach expanded in the wake of the scramble for Africa in the 1880s, more people visited or served or toured in the empire, and many returned ill or diseased. They included imperial servants, merchants, military personnel, missionaries, and tourists. For once, Manson's decision to pursue his career in the periphery for nearly two decades provided him with an advantage over his colleagues in Britain.

This was not the only irony in Manson's decision to relocate to London. He discovered malaria for the first time in his career. As the next chapter will show, the internationalization of malaria research spurred Manson's initial interest in the life history of the *Plasmodium* parasite. Laveran, the French surgeon in Algiers who had first drawn attention to the parasite as the cause of disease in 1878, directed Manson's interest to the role of the mosquito as intermediary. Unable to explain how the parasite left the human host, Laveran suggested the mosquito as a likely candidate, based on the analogy of Manson's flawed *filaria* worm research. Manson later made Laveran's hypothesis his own by recruiting Surgeon-Major Ronald Ross of the Indian Medical Service as a research collaborator and by creating a context for its discovery through the use of metropolitan publicity.

4
Making Imperial Science British Science
The Discovery of the Transmission of Malaria

AS Manson's work on the life cycle of the *filaria* worm shows, metropolitan cultural institutions, such as the library of the British Museum and the Victorian medical press, played a critical role in mediating the construction of knowledge about the empire. Still, it is important to appreciate that imperial medical science was not marked off from British science as qualitatively different. On the contrary, the very centrality of metropolitan institutions in making imperial science allowed its strategic representation as British science. A critical moment in this cultural transformation was the internationalization of the discovery of the *Plasmodium malariae* parasite as the cause of malaria disease.

By the time Manson returned to Britain in 1889, the cause of malaria had ceased being a research problem of the periphery. To be sure, skepticism greeted the 1880 discovery of "parasitic elements" in the blood by Alphonse Laveran in French colonial Algeria (Figure 9). Within a decade, however, there was hardly any question about the existence of the *Plasmodium malariae*. A research community, international in scope and dedicated to the study of the *plasmodium* parasite, rapidly emerged. Regular research coverage in the medical press in Europe and North America sustained this community and generated an even wider audience. International congresses institutionalized the *plasmodium* by providing frequent forums for presenting, debating, and shaping future research on the life cycle of the parasite.

Paradoxically, as knowledge of the *plasmodium* became internationalized, it became politicized in national terms. Interest in the *plasmodium* took place against the background of the rapid disintegration of political relations among the leading European powers after the 1880s. As national economies matured, competition among new and old nation-states intensified. The quest for new markets and sources of raw materials spurred imperial rivalries in Africa and Asia while simultaneously fanning the growth of domestic nationalism. In this context, the internationalization of the *plasmodium* did not diminish nationalism but, rather, provided another source of national competition in science.

To be sure, British scientists since the early nineteenth century had politicized science in national terms. When seeking state assistance and/or public support for research, Charles Babbage and others compared Britain unfavorably with continental rivals France and Germany.[1] The empire rarely, if at all, figured in their jeremiads on the inadequacy of public support for science. The international politics of the late nineteenth century made it possible to portray research about the empire as an expression of national science. As a source of national pride, then, the elaboration of the life history of the malaria parasite

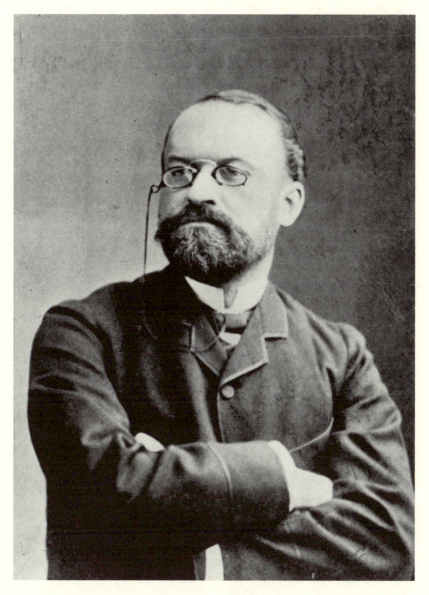

9. Alphonse Laveran, c. 1901. Photograph from the *Practitioner* (London), March 1901.

provided a space in which to recast the cultural meaning of British science. In a word, imperial science became British science.

This context both inspired Manson's research interest in the *plasmodium* parasite and facilitated the demonstration of the mosquito-malaria relationship. In 1891, Manson attended the Seventh International Congress of Hygiene and Demography in London, where Laveran was a featured presenter. Within the decade, Manson's name would be synonymous with the transmission of the *plasmodium* from mosquitoes to humans. In a December 1894 article in the *British Medical Journal*, Manson proposed that a suctorial insect might play a role in the life history of the malaria parasite outside the human bloodstream.[2] Before a British Medical Association meeting in Edinburgh four years later, he announced the effective demonstration of the transmission of the parasite to humans in the bite of the mosquito.[3]

At first glance, Manson's association with this discovery is surprising because of his location. Manson did not leave Britain, nor did he conduct any substantive research on the theory itself. Instead, Surgeon-Major Ronald Ross of the Indian Medical Service performed the time-consuming work over four years, largely independent of official support. It was Ross—not Manson—who demonstrated the mode of transmission in the bite of mosquitoes analogously in birds in the summer of 1898. Ironically, Ross made this discovery only after revising Manson's original theory, which stressed passive infection.

Yet, as metropolitan publicist for the mosquito-malaria theory, Manson played a decisive role in the process of discovery. Manson used the medical press and professional venues to generate an audience for the theory while Ross was engaged in its protracted demonstration. The wide gaps between Manson's public assertions and the verifiable evidence engendered skepticism at home and on the Continent. But criticism did not so much discredit the theory as create an audience for it. As I will show, Manson mobilized this audience. By portraying the mosquito-malaria theory as British science, he made support a question of patriotism and persuaded Indian authorities in Britain and India to facilitate its demonstration by placing Ross on special malarial research duty. This six-month assignment ultimately led to the discovery of the transmission of malaria in the bite of the mosquito.

The Internationalization of the Plasmodium Malariae

The *plasmodium* is not a worm but a single-celled protozoa.[4] It undergoes two cycles of replication: sporogony (the sexual cycle) and schizogony (the asexual

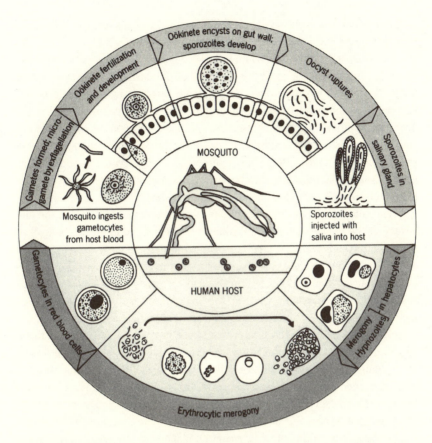

10. Life cycle of *Plasmodia vivax*. From Ralph Muller and John R. Baker, *Medical Parasitology* (London: Gower Medical Publications, 1990), 4.

cycle) (Figure 10). The female *Anopheles* mosquito introduces infective sporozoites into the human bloodstream during her blood meal. These spores migrate to the liver, where they develop and divide to become merozoites. After ten days, these merozoites enter the bloodstream and push through the cell membrane. As the red corpuscle closes in around it, the parasite presents the appearance of a pale hyaline spot. During cell division, the merozoite develops into the trophozoite, or "ring form," while displacing the hemoglobin by digesting it.

Once the corpuscle ruptures, new merozoites spill into the bloodstream and produce the telltale fever paroxysm in clinical malaria cases. (Depending on the reproductive cycle of the four common species of *plasmodia*, the paroxysm may occur every forty-eight or seventy-two hours.) Some merozoites develop into sexual forms. The conjugation of male and female gametocytes is essential to the completion of the life cycle of the parasite. Here the feeding habit of the female mosquito plays a crucial role. Once extracted from the bloodstream, some merozoites become macrogametes, the equivalent of the female ovum, while others become microgametes, which correspond to the spermatozoa. Zygotes, the offspring of these forms, enter the cells of the intestinal lining and develop into sporozoites. These sporozoites then migrate into the salivary glands of the mosquito. Once they have been injected into the bloodstream during the mosquito's next blood meal, the life cycle begins again.

The complex life cycle of the *plasmodium* parasite complicated the discovery of the cause of malaria. Without an understanding of the biology of sporozoa, investigators such as Laveran could only make informed guesses about the "parasitic elements" attached to corpuscles in the blood of malarial cases at the Constantine military infirmary in Algiers. These forms corresponded to the asexual phase and the beginning of the sexual phase. They included transparent hyaline forms, spheres with pigmented granules on the periphery and concentrated in a crown shape in the center as well as those with and without attached flagellum, and crescents with pigment in the center. Even though Laveran only superficially discussed the biological significance of these forms, the clinical evidence convinced him that the cause of malaria had been found. These "parasitic elements" were invariably present in febrile cases designated as malarial. Quinine—a chemotherapy long known as an antifebrile treatment—either eliminated or diminished their presence in the bloodstream.[5]

For all his conviction, Laveran was unable to do more than infer a causal relationship. He could not demonstrate the infectiousness of his "parasitic elements" experimentally. As a shortcut, Laveran could have injected infected blood into a healthy human subject. But, true to his convictions, he was unwilling to cause a needless death. Nor was bacteriology, the leading field of medical science, particularly helpful. The *plasmodium* parasite is an obligate parasite, one that requires at least two distinctive hosts (the *Anopheles* mosquito and the human bloodstream) to complete its life cycle. As Laveran learned from his attempts to cultivate the parasites in bacteriological cultures, exposure to the external environment simply killed them.[6]

Quite apart from Laveran's own limitations, there were other purported agents of malaria, chief among them was the *Bacillus malariae*. As early as 1874, Corrado Tommasi-Crudeli of Italy and Edwin Kelbs of Germany had identified a vegetable-based organism in water and soil samples from the Pontine region of Rome, an area notorious for malarial disease. Their evidence seemed incontrovertible.[7] They not only cultivated the organism and injected it into laboratory-bred rabbits but also produced the symptoms of malaria that were associated with human disease: persistently high temperatures and an enlarged spleen. The verification of the "microphyte or bacillus malaria" by other investigators entitled it, according to future U.S. surgeon-general George Sternberg, "to rank with spirium of relapsing fever, the anthrax bacillus, and the tubercle bacillus of Koch, among demonstrated germs."[8] At the International Medical Congress in Copenhagen in 1884, Tommasi-Crudeli sniffed at Laveran's forms, regarding them as little more than the by-products of deteriorating corpuscles caused by the presence of the *Bacillus malariae.*[9]

Laveran was not a little frustrated. He had made little headway since announcing the "parasitic elements." Since he could not demonstrate the infectiousness of his forms experimentally, he did so rhetorically, by analogy, in his 1884 treatise on malaria. "The parasites which are found in the blood of a patient stricken by intermittent fever are as characteristic of malaria as *trichina* is of *trichinosis*, or *filaria* is of *filariasis*. One still would be waiting for admitting to the rank of diseases parasites, *trichinosis* and *filariasis*, except that *trichina* and *filaria* have not been cultivated outside the organism." In stressing the infectious nature of the malarial parasite, Laveran posited a period of existence outside the human host. "At what state does the microbe of *paludism* live in the external environment, under what form and by what means are they introduced into our body?"[10]

Invoking the life cycle of the *filaria*, Laveran speculated that the malaria parasite underwent a form of alternative generation outside the human body, possibly in the mosquito. "The *filaria* embryoes which exist in the blood of patients stricken with *filariasis* are absorbed by the mosquitoes which suck the blood of the living, the *filaria* undergo a transformation in the body of the mosquitoes and when the last have died on the surface of standing water, the *filaria* escape in the water and are absorbed immediately with drinking water." Noting that mosquitoes were "abundant in all malaria localities," he rhetorically asked, "Do the mosquitoes play a role in the pathology of paludism as in the case of *filaria*?"[11] Laveran did not follow up this suggestion experimentally, but two Italian investigators, Giovanni Battista Grassi and Sauveur Calandruccio, did.[12] Their failure to detect evidence of morphological change would later become a source of skepticism about Manson's mosquito-malaria theory.

In the meantime, opinion about the existence of Laveran's parasite began to shift. By the time he published his treatise in 1884, the *Bacillus malariae* had been discredited.[13] Even Ettore Marchiafava and Angelo Celli, who had earlier doubted the existence of Laveran's parasite and confirmed the existence of the bacillus *malariae*, changed their minds and quickly appropriated the parasite.[14] Over the objection of Laveran, who feared being preempted, they designated the parasite *Plasmodium malariae*. Marchiafava and Celli pushed the pace of research by suggesting that the regular sequence of mutations of pigmented forms inside the corpuscle referred to the process of segmentation or asexual reproduction, common in the *sporozoa* family.[15]

It was left to Camillo Golgi of Pavia to elaborate the process of asexual reproduction in the bloodstream itself. In a series of articles in 1886, Golgi did more than simply describe the process of segmentation, that is, when the merozoites divided and ultimately ruptured the corpuscle. He also connected the fever cycle of malaria with the rupturing of the corpuscle. This observation clarified the meaning of the regularity of fevers in malaria disease and provided practitioners with an effective tool to diagnose disease. Golgi and other investigators ascribed the different febrile patterns of malaria disease to the replication cycles of different species of the *plasmodium* parasite: seventy-two hours for the quartan (*P. malariae*) and forty-eight for the tertian (*P. vivax*).[16]

The coverage of the *plasmodium* in the medical press in Europe and North America transformed Laveran's "parasitic elements" into an international phenomenon. Marchiafava and Celli placed their confirmation of Laveran's forms in the German journal *Fortschritt der Medicin*. Celli played host to Maj. George Sternberg in Rome during the summer of 1886 and made available malarial patients as well as laboratory facilities. When Sternberg returned to the United States, he published in the *Medical Record* a two-part lead article on the malarial parasite.[17] William Crookshank of King's College, London University, who had briefly studied at the Rome laboratory of Marchiafava, testified to the parasite's existence at the BMA meeting in 1887.[18] Dr. Romanovski, of St. Petersburg, reported that the parasite was consistently present in the blood of malarial cases.[19]

What a difference a decade made! Laveran's fame followed him to the Seventh International Congress on Hygiene and Demography in 1891 in London. This venue was a fortuitous one: it marked the first time Britain had hosted this congress since its inauguration in 1877. In the meantime, conflict shaped relations between British and continental approaches to public health especially in the wake of cholera visitations. British preference for urban sanitation over quarantine appeared to European hygienists to be not only self-serving for a trading nation but also hypocritical in light of the relative indifference to urban conditions in India. After being marginalized in previous congresses, the

Seventh Congress represented a vindication of British sanitary policy. As planning proceeded, the event quickly became an occasion to exhibit British science to the world. Queen Victoria agreed to serve as patron, and Edward, Prince of Wales, accepted the presidency of the Congress. "British presidents and other officers of Sections will be among the most eminent men in their several departments of knowledge," an editorial in *Nature* announced.[20] The rooms of the various natural science societies, housed in Burlington House, and of the University of London were made available for the twenty sections dedicated to presentations at the Congress.[21] As a model of sanitary science, the very nation would play host to the two thousand or more delegates who attended the Vienna Congress in 1887. It added, "It is anticipated that the Congress in London will attract at least an equal number of persons from foreign countries, because Great Britain affords so many examples of important sanitary works, as well as of institutions having the preservation or restoration of health as their main object."

In securing the participation of well over three thousand delegates from the Continent, British India, and other colonies, the Congress organizers furnished Laveran with an international stage.[22] None other than Sir Joseph Lister, Britain's elder statesman of medical science, presided at the bacteriological section, and investigators from the empire and the Continent were in attendance.[23] Savoring this occasion, Laveran did not offer any original research; rather, he chose to consolidate the evidence for the existence of the parasite. He noted that several investigators had confirmed the elements that he had first announced in 1880 and had suggested that there were more than two species of the parasite. Human-to-human inoculation experiments in Italy were reported to have produced the clinical symptoms of malaria in subjects. Further, the existence in birds of analogous endoglobular parasites, which resembled the pigmented elements and flagellated forms in other mammals, convinced Laveran that his parasite was specific to humans.[24]

Despite Laveran's confidence in the parasite as a causal agent, W. North, a former research scholar of the Grocers' Company, doubted the credibility of inoculation experiments in Italy, a region where malaria was believed to be endemic. "The only proof that organisms caused malaria was derived from experiments and inoculation, which [Laveran] maintained were valueless when performed in the country in which the malaria existed." Instead, North offered his own environmental, or "chill," theory, which described the disease as brought on by "the action upon the thermotoxic nervous system and by those violent changes from heat and cold which notoriously occur in all malarial countries."[25]

It was a sign of the credibility of the existence of the *Plasmodium* parasite that North's comments immediately elicited criticism. Neither Surgeon-
General Cook nor Ardasser V. Cooper, in their tours of service in India, could
adduce any evidence that climate caused or influenced malarial disease. Although the "chill theory" failed to convince the section, the *Plasmodium* was by
no means received as an unqualified scientific fact. Professor E. Crookshank of
King's College, University of London, acknowledged that Laveran's forms were
likely to be parasites and to be the cause of malaria. But Crookshank added
that the causal relationship was "not proved, and allied organisms were found
in healthy as well as in diseased animals." Laveran himself conceded that critical lacunae in knowledge of the life cycle of the parasite required illumination,
particularly the question of the form the parasite assumed outside the human
body and how it obtained access to the human host. He hoped that future comparative research on birds and other lower animals would furnish insight into
the life cycle of the malaria parasite in humans.[26]

Manson was present at the Congress. Two days before Laveran's presentation, he delivered a paper on the discovery of two new species of *filaria* in
central Africa.[27] Based on their common interest in parasites and mosquitoes,
one would think that Laveran and Manson would have sought each other out,
but a meeting between the two neither occurred nor was likely. Laveran was unaware that Manson was the discoverer of the mosquito's role as intermediary
host in the life history of the *filaria*. Nor did he discuss the mosquito's possible
role in his section paper.[28]

For his part, Manson had never detected Laveran's parasite. In China,
Manson had searched for the *Bacillus malariae*, shortly after the publication
of Laveran's first treatise in 1881 and later, when he moved to Hong Kong. In
neither attempt was he successful. By his own admission, he returned to Britain somewhat unsure about Laveran's parasite. "The consequence was that I
became somewhat sceptical about the value of Laveran's discoveries. Certain
it is that I returned to England without having seen or, at all events[,] having
recognised the parasite of malaria."[29]

Nonetheless, it is more than likely that Laveran made a strong impression on Manson. The discussion that followed his presentation undoubtedly impressed on Manson that though the life cycle of the parasite was incomplete, its
existence was not in doubt. The sensation created by Laveran inspired Manson
to turn to the *plasmodium* parasite in earnest. His timing could not have been
better. Even though the metropolitan press covered research developments,
relatively few investigators were studying the malarial parasite in Britain or in
the empire. Manson quickly filled this vacuum. Within two and a half years, he

had successfully used his location in London to establish himself as the most visible expert on the malarial parasite in Britain and the wider empire.

Cutting and Pasting: Manson and the Mosquito-Malaria Theory

Initially, practical difficulties prevented Manson from detecting the parasite himself. Until his appointment as visiting physician to the Branch Hospital of the Seamen's Hospital Society in May 1892, he did not have regular access to clinical malaria cases.[30] Even after this appointment, it took several months before he perfected the microscopic technique needed to detect the intracorpuscular stage of the parasite. Unlike the larger *filaria* helminth, the asexual malarial parasite occupies the cramped interior of the blood corpuscle. Exposing the corpuscle for microscopic detection was not an easy procedure for the uninitiated. When a blood drop, which consists of several spherical corpuscles, is placed on a flat surface, it assumes a *rouleaux* formation; that is, the edges of the corpuscles face the observer. Only by flattening the corpuscle, usually with the weight of the slip cover, could the observer see its interior. Patience was required in searching each slide for the pigmented forms; moreover, the presence of the asexual forms in the blood varied depending on the type of malaria infection.[31]

After a number of fruitless attempts, Manson reported success in the fall of 1893.[32] In a matter of months, he consolidated his position as the leading authority on the *plasmodium* parasite. He gave demonstrations on the microscopic identification of the *plasmodium* at the University College Hospital and the North London Medical and Chirurgical Society.[33] He published a malarial chart for the microscopic diagnosis of malaria in the *British Medical Journal* (Figure 11).[34] Manson's reputation was sufficiently well established that he not only served on the committee of adjudicators for the 1894 triennial Parkes Prize essay competition, whose topic was "Malarial Fevers: Their Causation and Prevention," but also chided the profession for its indifference to the malarial parasite.[35] During the 1894 annual oration before the Hunterian Society, Manson deplored the record of British science in this area.

It is little to our credit that continental nations, whose stake in tropical countries is infinitely smaller than ours, are nevertheless just as infinitely ahead of us in this matter; to them and to the Americans, all recent advances in our knowledge of malaria are due. England has wilfully, or, rather, ignorantly and indifferently, shut her eyes to one of the biggest facts in pathology revealed during the present century. We seem to have gone

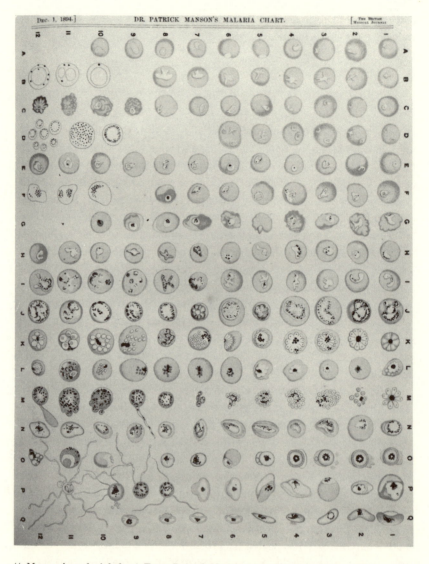

11. Manson's malarial chart. From *British Medical Journal*, 1 December 1894.

to sleep where we ought to have been hard at work and in the foremost ranks of the pioneers.[36]

Manson did not confine himself to transmitting knowledge about the *plasmodium* parasite. He soon focused on the very frontier of research: the life history of the *plasmodium* outside of the bloodstream. Although a consensus had formed about the asexual replication of the parasite in the bloodstream, there was considerable uncertainty about the meaning of the crescents (equivalent to gametocytes) and flagella (equivalent to microgametes) and their metamorphoses. Some investigators regarded the crescent as no more than the sterile, mature expression of the amoeboid form. Others, such as research collaborators Giovanni Grassi and R. Feletti, deemed it a distinctive new species of the malaria parasite.[37] Nor was there any more certainty about the flagellum. Because of its development from the crescent, Laveran had long viewed the flagellum as the most advanced form of the parasite. By contrast, Marchiafava and Celli rarely found free flagella in the peripheral blood of malarial patients, and the fact that the flagella tended to appear several minutes after the extraction of blood suggested to them the "appearance of agony" on exposure to the external environment.[38]

In one year's time, Manson's thinking about the meaning of these forms changed. In December 1893, he described the crescent as little more than a corpuscle folding on itself from the weight of the growing intracorpuscular bodies. "As for the flagellated bodies, I am at a loss to explain their position or role in the cycle of the parasite's life. . . . Undoubtedly, it belongs to the same organism as the extra- and intracorpuscular bodies; but what its exact relationship to these is I might conjecture, but could not say for certain."[39] A year later, Manson theorized that the crescent form was "intended to carry on the life of the species outside of the human body" and that the flagellum represented "the first stage in the life of the malaria organism outside the human body." The linchpin in the later life history of the malaria parasite, Manson continued, was a suctorial insect or mosquito.[40]

Manson's mosquito-malaria theory was a direct product of the internationalization of the discussion on the *plasmodium* parasite. Up to 1893, precious few extended treatises had been written on the *plasmodium* by British authors. Much of the important work had been published in French, German, or Italian. It is almost certain that Laveran's 1884 and 1892 treatises on malaria, in which he speculated on the role of the mosquito in the life history of the malarial parasite, remained largely unknown, or inaccessible, to Manson. This changed after the International Congress on Hygiene and Demography. The New Sydenham Society, a recently formed group dedicated to the diffusion of scientific research by foreign investigators, sponsored the translation of Laveran's 1891 treatise into English.[41] A year later the Society produced an English translation of Julius Mannaberg's comprehensive survey of *plasmodium* research up to 1893.[42] One reviewer of Laveran's treatise hoped that the volume would inspire greater interest in the subject of the malaria parasite.

We wonder how many of the men whose principal future lies in combating this organism have been brought face to face with the thing itself, have actually seen their future enemy, or been taught how to search for it. In this matter medical guides and teachers, both in this country and even in France itself, have a great deal to answer for. But signs of the recognition of the importance of Laveran's work are beginning to be discoverable. Evidence of this we have in the translation recently issued by the New Sydenham Society. We trust that this semi-official stamp of recognition will at last ensure its general acceptance by our countrymen, or at all events its thorough investigation.[43]

These two works inspired Manson to formulate the mosquito-malaria theory. Laveran's discussion of the epidemiology of the malaria parasite left a lasting impression on Manson. For the first time, Manson saw his work on the role of the mosquito in the life history of the *filaria* invoked as a basis for understanding the *plasmodium* outside the human bloodstream. As early as his 1884 treatise, Laveran had suggested that the mosquito might play a role in the life history of the *plasmodium* similar to its role in that of the *filaria*.[44] Although Laveran did not follow up this speculation experimentally, he provided collaborative evidence of the role of the mosquito as intermediary host in other infectious diseases in his later work. He volunteered a report about the work of Carlos Finlay, a Cuban physician, who had speculated that mosquitoes carried yellow fever. According to Dr. Bourel-Roncière, Timothy R. Lewis found twenty out of 140 female mosquitoes "filled with *filariae*." Laveran also cited a notice in the *Revue Scientifique* that swamp drainage in the United States led to a decline in malaria and "drove mosquitoes away." [45]

Laveran did not connect the role of the mosquito with the sequence of development of malarial forms, namely, the crescent and flagellum. This elision underscores Laveran's strategic deployment of a speculative epidemiology to buttress his claim of the infectiousness of his malarial parasite. Still, the implication of the connection between the malarial parasite and the mosquito was clear enough. He viewed the flagellum as the most advanced form of the parasite.[46] Unlike Laveran, Mannaberg was more explicit about the function of the crescent and the flagellum in the life history of the parasite outside the human bloodstream.

Mannaberg noticed distinct morphological changes in the parasite depending on whether he used a "dry" or "wet" mounting technique. The dry preparation was ideal for examining freshly drawn blood, because the interior of the blood corpuscles was preserved through the introduction of stain. While the dry technique offered a virtual snapshot of the contents of the blood in the body, it arrested the development of any vital forms. As a result, the forms of the crescent series such as fusiform ovals and spheres were rarely found, since they required twenty minutes or more to form outside the bloodstream. Conversely, wet mounting permitted the malarial forms to continue development at least until the blood was desiccated by excessive exposure to the air. Mannaberg inferred from the contrasting forms present in the different mounting techniques that the crescent form was associated with removal from the human body.

In perfectly fresh preparations very few fusiform or oval bodies are seen; therefore, as a rule, very few such bodies are seen in dry preparations which show the best condition of fresh blood. In consequence of this I incline to the idea that the alteration in form of the crescent is almost if not entirely coupled with its removal from the human body, and that the change never, or only rarely, occurs within the blood-vessels.[47]

Mannaberg's experience also shaped his perception of the function of the flagellum. Initially, he maintained that the flagellum was an intermediary stage that the parasite assumed in the soil, in what he called a "saprophytic condition," but his attempts to cultivate them to withstand this condition failed. Even the introduction of malarial blood "rich in spore-forming bodies or in crescents into animals" produced negative results, from which Mannaberg inferred that the malarial parasite required an animal or vegetable host outside the human body. "After all these unsuccessful attempts, it appears to be more and more probable that the malarial parasites do not exist in the external world as saprophytes, but must live as parasites either in animal or vegetable organisms."[48]

Together, Mannaberg and Lavern shaped the way Manson understood the future life history of the malarial parasite. Laveran suggested the mosquito as possible host; Mannaberg inferred that the crescent, and especially the flagellum, represented the protozoa's next stage of development outside the human host.[49] It took Manson little time to take the next deductive leap, concluding that the mosquito was the probable intermediary host of the malaria parasite. He admitted as much retrospectively in 1896. "It appeared to be that as neither Mannaberg nor Laveran had connected the mosquito with the flagellum, and . . . Calandruccio had failed to observe developmental changes in malarial parasites ingested by mosquitoes, the logic of the situation had been missed."[50]

Manson's most significant contribution in the making of the mosquito-malaria theory lay in framing the existence of the parasite outside the blood-stream as a biological necessity. In the opening of his 1894 article, Manson appealed to the biology of malaria disease to establish its infectious nature. Echoing Golgi, he noted, "The presence of this parasite in the blood precedes and accompanies a special type of fever; the cycle of its development coincides in the main with the cycle of the fever; and it disappears from the blood with spontaneous recovery from or cure the fever." [51] While the presence of the parasite in the bloodstream was indicative of malarial illness, its presence was temporary.

Manson buttressed the case for the excorporeal stage of the malaria parasite with a speculative epidemiology that was suspiciously close to Laveran's reasoning. Just as Laveran insisted that the parasite was infectious but not contagious, Manson noted, "Apart from communication by transfusion of blood, the malaria organism and malarial diseases can be acquired only indirectly either through air, the water, by food, or by other unknown way." Just as Laveran's failure to find his pigmented forms in the external environment induced him to speculate on the possibility of an alternative host, Manson cited the existence of malaria where humans were absent as further presumptive evidence of an excorporeal stage. "As it has been shown that the malaria organism is not directly communicable (in a normal way) by one individual to another, that it can be acquired in places where there is no human population, it follows that it has a second life, one outside and independent of the human body." [52]

Next, Manson underscored the temporary nature of the blood as a habitat for the malaria parasite by describing its development inside and outside the bloodstream. Here, too, previous investigators had used similar reasoning for a putative excorporeal stage of the parasite. Manson reported that the ubiquitous pigmented parasite underwent little development while in the bloodstream; to be sure, it changed form from oblong or oval to spherical, but it did not adopt any distinctive characteristics or physiological differentiation. The crescents remained in the bloodstream even after the fever had passed, either spontaneously or due to the action of quinine. Phagocytes, the body's immunological defensive agents, did not attack the crescent forms. Nor did these forms leave the body through the normal evacuation of fluids. Manson declared that the crescents remained passive as long as they remained in blood corpuscles. [53]

It was the generation of flagellated forms from the crescent that convinced Manson that the malarial parasite required a further extracorporeal stage of development. He noticed that extracted blood, when permitted to sit for several minutes, produced flagellated bodies from crescents. These bodies, as well as free flagella, appeared along the membrane of the crescent after a series of mutations from oblong or oval to spherical. Manson regarded even flagella that were generated from the intracorpuscular bodies as "analogous to the crescentic bodies, and on the same grounds as bodies destined for the continuation of the species."[54]

Once Manson had established the epidemiological and biological necessity for an excorporal stage, he rhetorically asked what was the nature of "this extraneous agent which assists the malaria to escape from the human body." To support the role of an insect host, Manson, like Laveran, invoked the analogy of the *filaria*. Like the *filaria* embryo, the *plasmodium* was parasitic and circulated in the bloodstream; it was not evacuated in the normal body fluids. The blood corpuscle protected the malaria parasite from phagocytes just as the sheath that enclosed the *filaria* embryo prevented it from leaving the bloodstream. Experimentation demonstrated that the evolutionary processes of both parasites commenced once they were removed from the bloodstream. The parallels between the two parasites convinced Manson that the mosquito, or a similar suctorial insect, was the host of the malaria parasite.

As the problem and conditions are the same for both organisms, the solution of the problem may also be the same for both. If this be the case, the mosquito having been shown to be the agent by which filaria is removed from the human blood vessels, this, or a similar suctorial insect, must be the agent which removes from the human blood vessels those forms of the malaria organism which are destined to continue the existence of this organism outside the body. It must, therefore, be in this or in a similar suctorial insect or insects that the first stages of the extracorporeal life of the malaria organisms are passed.[55]

Manson made some effort to demonstrate the theory himself. He solicited support from the British Medical Association as well as from the Royal Society for a research expedition to Demerara in the West Indies. But the latter denied his application, and the former only awarded him £150.[56] However, even if Manson had received funding, it is unlikely that he could have demonstrated the theory. Since his China days, he had suffered from recurring bouts of gout that left him debilitated for days. A trip abroad would further compromise his health; moreover, he simply could not financially afford to be away from his fledgling practice. The chance visit of Ronald Ross to his home made a research visit to the West Indies unnecessary (Figure 12).

Until 1892, when interest in Laveran's parasite began to spread among Anglo-Indian workers, Ross briefly speculated that malaria resulted from intestinal poisoning. He did not know how to search for or detect the malarial parasite. But Ross was sufficiently expert as a microscopist to expose a num-

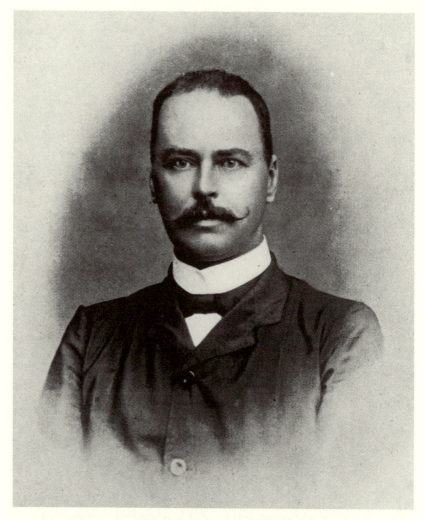

12. Ronald Ross, c. 1908. From Ronald Ross, *Memoirs, with a Full Account of the Great Malaria Problem and Its Solution* (London: John Murray, 1923).

ber of instances in which workers had confused the normal appearances in the blood with the purported parasite.[57] Ross's furlough to Britain coincided with the Parkes Prize essay competition on the cause and prevention of malarial fevers. During the early months of 1894, Ross read the literature on malaria at the library of the British Museum and consulted with Professor Kanthack, a pathologist at his former medical school at St. Bartholomew's Hospital.[58]

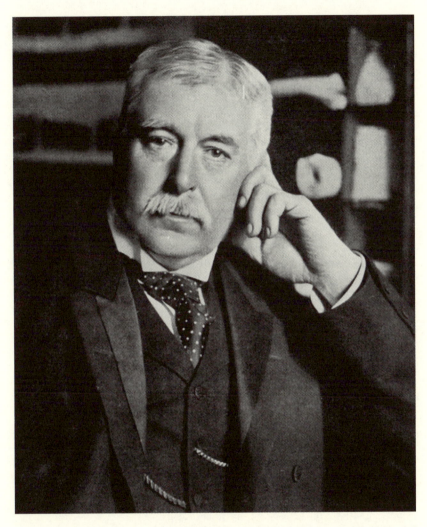

13. Patrick Manson, c. 1905. From Philip H. Manson-Bahr and A. Alcock, *The Life and Work of Sir Patrick Manson* (London: Cassell, 1927).

Kanthank confirmed the existence of the *plasmodium* and recommended that Ross visit Manson, the leading authority on the subject in Britain (Figure 13).[59]

When Ross called, Manson was out. But the visit was a pleasant surprise. Manson was familiar with Ross from his articles in the *Indian Medical Gazette* on the erroneous detection of the *plasmodium*.[60] Even though Ross had not independently detected the malarial parasite, Manson was impressed with his skill in microscopy. He also saw an opportunity to recruit a potential research collaborator. Manson offered his assistance to Ross: "I am certain, judging from the minuteness and accuracy of your observations, that you have not seen the *plasmodium malariae*, otherwise you would never have failed to recognise its pathological character. And the reason you have not seen it is the technique you employ. It will give me great pleasure to be of any service to you, for I am quite sure you can do the work and have patience to do it."[61] When Ross later returned, Manson showered attention on him. Manson revealed the malarial parasite in dry and wet preparations. "Within a few minutes," Ross recalled, "he showed me the Laveran's bodies which are technically called 'crescents' in a stained specimen of malaria blood. My doubts were now removed; and in a few days Manson demonstrated the other forms at Charing Cross Hospital and also took me on several occasions, with great kindness, to the Seamen's Hospital (at Royal Albert Dock in East London)."[62]

Ross soon became a regular visitor to Manson's home. During his visits, Manson shared with him the latest works by Laveran, Mannaberg, and others. In doing so, Manson gave Ross a leg up on the competition for the Parkes Prize essay competition, which he later won. These books, as well as the two men's discussions (undoubtedly about the extracorporeal function of the crescent and flagellum forms), created a context in Ross's mind for the plausibility of the mosquito-malaria theory. A month before the publication of his theory, Manson confided in Ross. "I have formed a theory," Ross recalled Manson saying during their walk down Oxford Street, "that mosquitoes carry malaria just as they carry *Filariae*." Ross was more than impressed; he was "determined to test the hypothesis thoroughly on [his] return to India."[63] He said as much in his prize-winning essay.

The inference is very clear. Dr. Manson thinks that as soon as the blood cools in the stomach of the second host, the crescent and large spherical bodies put forth the curious flagella and undergo a rhabditic stage; and the argument appears extremely cogent to me. What animal harbors the parasite is of course a subject for the most interesting investigation. . . . A number of possibilities suggest themselves to me, which it is unnecessary to mention until I shall have had an opportunity of testing them; in the meantime however the form of the parasite gives much presumptive evidence.[64]

Ross was not drawn to the mosquito-malaria theory by Manson's charisma alone. He needed to advance his stalled career. He had little to show for nearly fifteen years of service. Before Ross met Manson, he had held only one permanent position.[65]

Ross's career was not an anomaly but a matter of course for the IMS. Following the Indian Mutiny in 1857, Britain's presence in India expanded. The number of doctors grew to meet the health needs of imperial personnel and colonial charges in times of peace and war. There was no corresponding growth in the number of permanent positions, however. This imbalance, together with a strict adherence to seniority, reduced medical personnel to long waits for secure positions, broken up by temporary assignments. For Ross, the demonstration of the malaria-mosquito relationship offered a once-in-a-lifetime opportunity to transform his fortunes with a dazzling discovery. He therefore returned to India motivated to change his fortunes through the malaria parasite.

"Follow the Flagellum!"—Discovery Through Publicity

The approach that Manson and Ross adopted to demonstrate the hypothesis experimentally was built on a false premise, namely, that the flagellum bored through the cellular lining of the mosquito and developed into an unknown form. Based on this premise, all that Ross required were mosquitoes and clinical cases infected with the *plasmodium*. By subjecting the patients to mosquito bites, he hoped to reveal evidence of vital development in the abdomen of the mosquito, namely, the metamorphosis of the crescent, flagellated spore into the flagellum. From here, the task grew increasingly difficult. Beyond the distinctive pigmentation associated with the intracorpuscular stage of the *plasmodium*, Ross's search in the body cavity of the mosquito amounted to looking for a needle in a haystack. He not only had to master the physiology and anatomy of the mosquito and distinguish other parasites of the mosquito but also had to isolate the unknown form of the *plasmodium*.

Leaving his wife and two children in London, Ross returned to Secunderabad to join his regiment, the Nineteenth Madras Infantry, in April 1895. With only routine duties, he immediately turned his attention to establishing the adaptive relationship between the mosquito and the *plasmodium*.[66] Establishing this relationship involved comparing the development of parasite forms extracted from the finger blood of infected humans (or his control subjects) with the blood expelled from mosquitoes that fed on infected humans. By showing that the sequence of development from crescent, spheroids, and flagellate bodies occurred faster in the mosquito, Ross hoped to show that the mosquito was a likely natural host for the *plasmodium*.

Within a matter of weeks, Ross reported encouraging results.

I got a ½ mosquito and *smeared* his blood with the needle on cover glass, inverted the same after drying in air and simply laid on slide. . . . *Nothing but spherules*. Not a single crescent and only one or two masses of spent pigment (?). A control finger blood made in same way gave, of course, *all crescents and no spherules*; while a finger blood, which

had been kept for two hours and was then opened and dried, gave *mostly crescents &*
a few spherules. . . . This last experiment then seems to me to prove that the crescents
undergo change into spherules in the stomach of the mosquito as outside; and to *suggest*
that they do so faster than in control specimens.[67]

Ross gave life to Manson's theory. "The mere fact that the parasite is not
digested is enough to prove to my mind that it is in its proper habitat, and the
fact you have discovered that it advances in development more rapidly and
more frequently in the mosquito's stomach is confirmatory of this inference."
The timing of Ross's letter could not have been better. Manson had planned to
discuss the life history of the parasite at the July meeting of the British Medical Association in London. Manson now saw an opportunity to present visual
evidence of the development of the parasite in the mosquito seven months after
publishing his theory. Appealing to Ross's self-interest, Manson asked for slide
preparations of exflagellation. "If I was armed with a series of such preparations I could speak with authority of your work which could not be controverted
and you may be sure that I will give you a good shove and help you as far as I
can to the ear of authorities in India who may be in a position to forward your
investigations."[68]

A week after his early detection of crescent-spherical-flagella development, Ross tested these results by wet blood smears alone. He examined the
abdomens of some twenty hand-cultivated mosquitoes that had fed on the same
malarial blood over a period of several days. Ross found greater and greater
numbers of spherules, many exhibiting eruptive movement, a find that reinforced his suggestion that the abdomen was the natural site for the parasite.
After several attempts, Ross finally detected flagella in fields with spherules.
Additional examinations convinced him: "I am inclined on the whole, after examining 28 mosquitoes, to gather that the stomach of the mosquito is very probably the natural *locus* for the crescent-spherule-flagella metamorphosis."[69]

After these results, Ross was particularly eager to confirm the main outlines of Manson's hypothesis. He closed his letter to Manson with a description
of a human passive-infection experiment. "Presently I shall give infected mosquitoes, and the water they have died in, to natives on payment and see results;
then for seeing where the flagella go."[70] By adopting this approach, Ross took a
shortcut. A positive infection experiment would buttress Manson's belief in the
hypothesis and at the same time reinforce his efforts to follow the intercellular
development of the flagellum in the mosquito.

As much as Manson wanted to impress the audience at the BMA meeting,
the occasion proved to be a disappointment.[71] Ross could not provide the preparations in time; his supply of mosquitoes and infected human cases dried up.[72]

As it turned out, there was little that was original in Manson's presentation. Besides describing the appearance of the *plasmodium* in the human blood-stream, Manson could only describe Ross's observations on parasite development in the mosquito. "This observer [Ross]," according to a *Lancet* account of the proceedings, "has found that the parasites are able to resist destruction in the stomach of this insect, and passing thence into the blood occur much more frequently in the flagellate form than in blood drawn from the finger of a patient with malaria; its development in the intermediate host is also evidenced by the fact that the crescent forms all become spheres." Manson cited one of Ross's successful passive-infection experiments as further evidence of the role of the mosquito to buttress his claim of the passive mode of infection. "He explained the communication of the disease from insect to man by supposing that the parasites on the death of the mosquito are added to water or soil, and by that means are carried into the human body."[73]

George Thin, who was familiar with Manson's work on the *filaria* worm, was not satisfied with Manson's presentation of the mosquito-malaria relationship. Although Thin concurred with the notion that the malarial parasite was probably transmitted passively in water, he questioned the role of the mosquito. He drew "attention to the fact that in Sierra Leone . . . malarial fever is very common, but mosquitoes are rare." In reply, Manson could only retreat to his conviction that the parasite "must have some third form not yet discovered."[74] In a letter to Ross, Manson sniped at Thin: "I don't know when the *BMJ* will publish my paper on your work. I suppose soon. The accounts given it, as usual, are inaccurate. Thin tried to throw cold water on it, but the feeling of the meeting was distinctly in its favour—not that that makes any difference to the facts. The merry microbe goes its own way regardless of what people do and say about it."[75]

Seven months later, the subject of the mosquito-malaria theory surfaced again at other professional meetings. The first was a meeting of the Royal Medical and Chirurgical Society, where George Thin and his coauthor, Robert Marshall, discussed the malarial parasite in Spain. Based on the epidemiology of malaria in Spain, Thin reiterated his doubts about the role of the mosquito. "The facts supported the conclusion come to by the Italian authorities that drinking water was not the usual medium by which poison was conveyed, and they were strongly against the theory suggested by Laveran, Pfeiffer, and others, that mosquitoes or other insects might act the part of an intermediate host." Dr. Curnow, a visiting physician at the Seamen's Hospital Society, agreed that "the hypothesis that mosquitoes acted as an intermediate host was not proved."[76]

Manson apparently was not present at this meeting. But a week and a half

later, he drew attention to his theory during a discussion of another paper by
Thin on the microscopic appearances in the tissue of a fatal case of pernicious
malaria in Sierra Leone. Hoping to distance himself from experiments by Giovanni Battista Grassi and Sauveur Calandruccio that had earlier cast doubt
on Laveran's suggestion, Manson "disclaimed any connection with Laveran's
mosquito theory." As he had not done on previous occasions, he fortified his
biological inferences, which made the mosquito a candidate for intermediary
host, with slides of sectioned mosquitos containing parasites. These poorly preserved slides, which Manson received after his BMA presentation, did not impress anyone. Dr. Galloway warned that "any dogmatic statements about the
life-history and stages of the malarial parasite are likely to impede advance"
and offered the life cycle of the discredited coccidium oviforme as a caution-
ary example. Thin remained "an agnostic" on the hypothesis. He "did not deny
the possibility of its truth but all proof was wanting. Hypotheses were useful
private guides for work, but facts were wanted, not theories."[77]

It is tempting to portray the skepticism about the theory as the obtuse con-
servatism of the British medical profession. But more than a year after publishing his theory, Manson had not demonstrated the role of the mosquito. Without a
comprehensive understanding of the sexual stage of the *plasmodium*, it is unlikely that well-preserved slide sections of the metamorphosis of the crescent-
sphere-flagellum series would have been any more persuasive than a speculative description of the life history of the protozoa. Manson wanted medical men
to believe in the mosquito-malaria theory based on little more than his word.
Actually, Thin's reluctance showed considerable restraint.

The slow pace of verification frustrated Manson as well. In September
1895, Ross was placed on cholera duty in Bangalore, suspending research until
the spring of 1896. More than ever, Manson was eager for slides; he had agreed
to give the Goulstonian lectures at the Royal College of Physicians in March
1896. "I am anxious to be able to demonstrate in a convincing manner to sneer-
ing sceptics that the crescent does really undergo change in the mosquito and
I would fain hope that by studying sections of the mosquito stomach in series
we may be able to trace the progress of the flagella after they have broken
away." Enclosing a box of small bottles containing formaline, Manson pressed
for specimens. "My lectures are in March and I would therefore have to be hard
at work all February or earlier if possible. You would therefore require to have
the box or some specimens despatched so as to reach me by that time. Any expense you may be put to on my account please send me a note of. Perhaps you
could contrive to send me a few mosquitoes in the course of a mail or two."[78]

The wait for the parcel from India must have been an emotional rollercoaster for Manson. Ross did not reply until late November and feared that his cholera duty assignment might prevent him from preparing slides, much less devoting his energies to the elaboration of the theory.[79] In December, he managed to dispatch twelve infected mosquitoes. Relieved, Manson wrote, "I shall welcome the twelve apostles—I mean the twelve mosquitoes in glycerine for I hope to make them apostles in a malaria sense—preachers of the gospel of Laveran and of the cause you and I have at heart." [80]

By January 1896, Manson's anxiety had returned. The "twelve apostles" had not arrived and the time before his lectures was fast evaporating. "I have been hoping to send you an account of the results of my examination of those twelve glycerine mosquitoes which in your letter of 3rd December you said you had sent off to me. But the infernal things have never turned up and I am in despair about concluding my Goulstonian Lectures fearing that the bottle has miscarried or come to grief somehow." He gently prodded Ross: "Would you ask at your post office and if you have one or two malariated insects ready, on receipt of this they might yet be in time if sent off at once via Brindisi. The first lecture is on the 10th of March; and the second not until the 17th I think. They are likely to be published soon after delivery and I shall try to send you an advance proof before." [81]

While waiting for the arrival of Ross's parcel, Manson deferred the discussion of the process of exflagellation in the mosquito in his lectures as long as he could. It is for this reason that the first two lectures largely represented an elaboration on his 1894 article and a description of Ross's 1895 observations on exflagellation.[82] By the time of the second lecture, Manson decided to gamble, hoping that Ross's mosquitoes would arrive in time for the third lecture. This was risky, since the mosquitoes would have to be sectioned, stained, and mounted. In his second lecture, Manson acknowledged that he did not know where the parasite made its home in the cellular structure of the mosquito, but he raised expectations by implying that it would be known shortly.

Perhaps, owing to the minuteness of the objects we are dealing with and the many practical difficulties attending the investigation, it may be long before that cell is found, and the full history of the parasite in the mosquito thoroughly worked out; but I feel certain that these things will be established in time, and on the lines I indicate, and that the life-history of the plasmodium will be revealed as completely for the mosquito as it already has been for man.[83]

The "twelve apostles" did not arrive in time for the third lecture. Disappointed and probably not a little embarrassed, Manson complained about the "vagaries of the Indian parcel post." "Had the malariated mosquitos . . . arrived," he offered, "I believe I could have demonstrated to you the flagellum *en route* to its cells and, possibly, the developing flagellum actually lying in the cell itself." Without slide preparations, the high point of the lecture was decidedly anticlimactic. Manson was reduced to illustrating the "first step"—the sequence of flagellum development in the mosquito, or exflagellation—not with slides but with drawings.[84]

Even Manson acknowledged the inadequacy of his presentation. To those critics, such as George Thin, who had chided Manson for publishing before having the facts, he conceded, "I ought to have waited for the advance which I so confidently anticipate[d] before communicating such results as have already been arrived at in this matter of demonstrating the plasmodium in the mosquito. I feel that there is a certain amount of ground for such criticism." Nonetheless, he defended his actions on the grounds that publicity was essential to scientific investigation:

At the same time, I would plead that progress is favoured by publicity, that the co-operation of many workers is necessary, or at least desirable, in this as in all similar inquiries. It may be that someone, more fortunately situated as regards material and opportunity than either Ross or myself, may, by the publication of what has already been done, have his attention drawn to this line of investigation, and so be led to advance the inquiry still further, and perhaps, happily, to the completion of our work.[85]

Amico Bignami, a professor of pathology at Rome University and a leading malaria investigator, was not particularly impressed by Manson's Goulstonian lectures.[86] Bignami was not opposed to the hypothesis. On the contrary, he found Laveran's epidemiological reasoning plausible and even suggested the possibility of the transmission of the parasite in the bite of the mosquito, rather than passively as Manson had speculated.[87] What Bignami objected to was Manson's scientific style, his use of rhetorical devices to buttress his arguments.[88] He took exception to Manson's a priori assumption that the *plasmodium* required an excorporeal stage.

This conviction, founded on arguments drawn from analogy, leads the lecturer to inquire how the plasmodium escapes from the human body; for granting his sequence of ideas, this becomes one of the fundamental questions. Considering *a priori* the escape as necessary, he does not ask if this happens as a rule, but only how it happens; and takes this inquiry as a starting-point for the study of the malarial parasite in outer nature.[89]

Nor was Bignami persuaded by Manson's argument regarding the function of the flagella as the analogue to the malaria spore in the human body. "The flagellate body would thus be a parasite in the state of sporulation, 'whose spores in the interests of the extracorporeal life of the plasmodium' take this special form. It is easy to oppose to this the fact that the flagella do not contain chromatin and have the aspect and the structure of simple protoplasmic filaments. How then can they be looked upon as spores?" Bignami implied that without an adequate appreciation of the function of the flagellum or its relationship to the life cycle of the parasite, Ross's observations of accelerated flagellation in the stomach of the mosquito did not constitute a demonstration of the "first step."[90]

Manson relished the attention from Bignami; any publicity was good publicity. After the disappointment of his Goulstonian lectures, Bignami's criticism indicated that investigators on the Continent were beginning to take notice of the mosquito-malaria theory. "I do not send the letter as there is no saying how soon I may have to refer to it now that attention is being directed in Italy and France to this matter of the mosquito in Malaria," Manson wrote to Ross. Manson intimated that he intended to reply to Bignami: "Bignami has criticised our theory in *Il Policlinico* and has started a mosquito theory of his own. . . . Bignami is wrong in many things and blinks all my arguments nearly. I propose to answer him as soon as the paper appears."[91]

Manson published his reply two months later. "Emanating from so eminent an authority this criticism presumably includes everything of importance adducible against these views. Though not altogether favourable the remarks have strengthened rather than weakened my convictions as to the special *role* I attribute to the mosquito in the malaria drama." Rather than offering substantive evidence to support the a priori function of the flagellum, Manson instead attacked Bignami's critique by engaging in semantics. "I do not, as Bignami represents, say that movement is a proof of life; I merely say that movement is one of the evidences of life. But I do give it to be inferred that complex movements of protoplasm, such as the malaria flagellum exhibits, amount to a proof of life." Regarding the presence of a nucleus in the flagellum, Manson challenged Bignami's authorities: "Would Bignami enumerate the observers who have themselves actually endeavored seriously to work at this point and say how many attempts they have made and how they set about making these attempts?" Without denying the presence of the nucleus, Manson conceded that he had not seen it: "It is a difficult and very rare thing to get the flagellated body in a condition suitable for staining in such a way as to render any nucleus it may contain visible."[92]

In the meantime, Ross's cholera assignment in Bangalore was due to end in the spring of 1896. He was loath to return to his regimental post. Research materials, that is, mosquitoes and clinical cases, were hard to get. Ross, too, believed that he was entitled to a much better situation than a mere "native" regiment. But six months of pushing for a better appointment had failed. He had hoped to snag a staff-surgeoncy in Bangalore or the rumored special appointment under E. H. Hankin, the government chemical examiner at Agra, but both either fell through or did not materialize.[93] Ross even lobbied Madras officials to subsidize a malarial research expedition to the Nilghiri Hills of Ootacamund. Though Madras granted him two months' privilege leave, the government of India was not prepared to underwrite the expedition. Resigned to his fate, in April 1897 Ross hired servants and went out to Ootacamund for three months.[94]

Ross came down with malaria; otherwise, his expedition was largely uneventful. He made no headway with the theory.[95] Up to this point, he had complained about his stalled career while soldiering on as best he could. Manson responded with words of encouragement and tried to use his personal relationships in the India Office to secure for Ross special malaria duty or any appointment, but without success.[96] After the failed expedition, Ross's complaints turned into threats of resignation. "The fact is that in spite of all my work and frequent official commendation, I now hold what may be described as the worst appointment in the Service, namely medical charge of a native regiment; and so far as I see I should continue to hold it and not get anything better were I to do as much and as good scientific work as yourself, Laveran, Lewis, etc., etc. put together." [97]

Manson could ill afford to lose Ross. No one else had volunteered to demonstrate the mosquito-malaria theory. Concerned about an indefinite halt to research, Manson directly solicited the assistance of Charles Crosthwaite, undersecretary for India. In forwarding Ross's request for a special posting at a planned pathological institute in Madras, Manson appealed to Crosthwaite's sense of patriotism. "We are cutting a sorry figure alongside other nations in this matter just at present," Manson complained. "To our national shame be it said just few, very few of the wonderful advances in the science of the healing art which have signalised recent years, have been made by our countrymen. It is particularly apparent in the matter of tropical diseases which we should in virtue of our exceptional opportunities be facile princeps." [98]

For Manson, the demonstration of the mosquito-malaria theory offered an opportunity to "rehabilitate our national character and to point out to the rest of the world how to deal with the most important disease." Manson warned that if Ross was not given the opportunity to pursue the hypothesis, Britain again risked embarrassment: "If we dont do it and do it soon, some Italians or Frenchmen or Americans will step in and show us how to do what we cant or wont do for ourselves. They are on the track even now." In a final appeal for the hypothesis, Manson asked, "Can you influence the powers that be at the India Office to give Ross the chance of striking a good stroke for England? He asks for little and may do a very great deal indeed."[99]

Manson's appeal to Crosthwaite came at a fortuitous time. Since 1894, the Anglo-Indian medical profession had been stewing over the public flogging delivered to it by Ernest Hart, the crusading and enterprising editor of the *British Medical Journal*. In a speech before the Indian Medical Congress, Hart deplored the menial duties that medical officers were required to perform and denounced official hostility to research. It was no wonder that the profession in India had done little to advance the understanding of the *plasmodium*: "It is a somewhat strange circumstance that, although we have been acquainted with this parasite now for some fourteen years, and although many pathologists in Italy, in France, in Germany, and in America have occupied themselves with its study, it has been entirely, or almost entirely, neglected by the profession in India and England."[100]

Indian authorities in Britain and India had weathered similar broadsides for nearly half a century.[101] But Manson made Crosthwaite's decision relatively easy. Ross did not require much, just a better situation. The political windfall that would result from the demonstration of the theory seemed worth a few well placed letters. Shortly after Manson's entreaty, Crosthwaite consulted with W. R. Hooper, president of the India Office Medical Board (1895–1903). Using his knowledge of the availability of civilian appointments, Hooper recommended that Ross apply in person for a civil appointment in the Central Provinces, preferably for Jabalpore. To facilitate Ross's appointment, Crosthwaite furnished him with a letter of introduction to J. P. Hewitt, the provincial secretary, whom he knew. He also volunteered to visit Lord Hamilton, the secretary of state for India, and to forward Manson's letter to Lord Elgin, the viceroy.[102] Even though Crosthwaite cautioned that appointments were decided by "Indian authorities," Manson expected that the Indian Medical Service would "fix" Ross shortly.[103]

While Crosthwaite worked on Ross's behalf, Manson turned up the heat under Indian officials. A notice in the *British Medical Journal*, which undoubtedly originated from Manson, reported that Ross had sacrificed his health in the service of medical science while in the jungles of India. "We regret to learn that Surgeon-Major Ronald Ross, I.M.S., who has been employing three months' leave in investigating the malaria mosquito theory, has unfortunately contracted the infection upon which he was endeavouring to throw light." In a blunt appeal, Manson expressed hope that Ross would be rewarded for his labors: "We trust that the devotion which he has shown in the cause of medical science and humanity will have a better reward than a dose of jungle fever, and that every facility will be granted to enable him to bring his disinterested and arduous labors to a satisfactory conclusion and with as little danger to his health as possible." [104]

The lobbying activity, together with Ross's own persistence, appeared to work. The secretary to Leslie Cleghorn, the director-general of the Indian Medical Service (1895–97), alerted Ross that a civil surgeoncy in the Central Provinces was likely to be offered to him shortly.[105] Writing from Secunderabad in late July, Ross exclaimed, "The only adequate thanks I can give you is to solve the problem!" [106] Ross knew what he had to do. "I see my course clearly now—it is to make an exhaustive search on these lines. I shall not miss a cytozoon, a spore, an amoeba, or a flagellum, believe me. When the brindled mosquitoes are done with I will try another species. The animal will be found if it is there, which it must be." [107]

From July through August, Ross hunted for the flagellum in earnest while awaiting news of his expected appointment. His method consisted of concurrent mosquito-feeding experiments. One group of mosquitoes fed on malaria cases; a second group fed on normal blood. By comparing the cellular structures, Ross hoped to identify the next stage of the *plasmodium* in the tissue of the mosquito. Through a frustrating process of elimination, Ross determined that brown mosquitoes, rather than brindled mosquitoes, were more accommodating hosts. The cellular linings of the intestines of infected brown mosquitoes revealed pigmentation.[108] Ross quickly forwarded his findings to the *British Medical Journal* and his slide preparations to Manson.[109]

Ross's detection was the first substantive news that Manson had received in nearly two years. When asked by Ernest Hart about the significance of Ross's submission, Manson urged immediate publication.[110] In fact, Manson wrote the lead article in the *British Medical Journal*. He hoped that the article would "give the friends you have a handle to work with in attempts on the Indian Government." [111] The article emphasized that Thin, John Bland-Sutton, and Manson had confirmed Ross's observations of cells containing melanin, a product associated with the parasite. Further research was necessary to determine whether the presence of these pigmented cells indicated the biological development of the malaria parasite or was simply a by-product of the contents of the mosquito's stomach. "The settlement of this question is of the highest scientific and practical importance." [112]

Manson was hopeful that Ross's "devotion, persistency, and ability . . . will . . . be rewarded with a discovery not less important to humanity than that Laveran's discovery itself, which would be a fitting complement [*sic*]." In a direct appeal to the Indian authorities and to British national pride, Manson pleaded "in the interest of British biological and medical science, that every opportunity will be afforded Dr. Ross to prosecute his investigations under favourable conditions, for they are investigations which may be pregnant with benefit to mankind, investigations which nothing should be allowed to hamper." Otherwise, better-subsidized French or German investigators would reap what British science had sowed.[113]

Manson also orchestrated several endorsements, including his own, which were attached as an addendum to Ross's article. Without declaring that the pigmented forms were related to the *plasmodium*, Manson came close to it:

There can be no question that these cells contain pigment optically indistinguishable from the pigment which is so characteristic a feature in the malaria parasite. . . . Considering the peculiar grouping of the pigment in many instances, a grouping that forcibly recalls what one sees in the living malarial parasite, and the distinctness and regularity of the outlines of the bodies, I am inclined to think Ross may have found the extracorporeal phase of malaria.[114]

Ross's slide preparations convinced Thin, who had doubted the theory for over three years. Manson wrote to Ross that now Thin "recognised their likeness to the malaria parasite and the importance of your find."[115] Even though Thin did not regard the pigmented forms as conclusive evidence of plasmodium development per se, he was so impressed that he urged that Ross's work continue.

It is . . . very important that Surgeon-Major Ross, with his exceptional capacity and opportunities, should continue his investigations not only regarding the mosquito in connection with the parasite of malaria, but also by working in any other lines which his observations point out to him as possibly leading to a solution of the unsolved riddle of the existence of the parasite outside the human body, for outside the human body we know it does and must exist.

Like Manson, Thin concluded with an appeal for more resources for Ross's research: "In the interests of science it is therefore most desirable that support, assistance if required, and every facility should be given to him to enable him to continue his researches."[116]

Ross's prospects only appeared to be improving: The promised appointment never materialized. Worse was to follow: War broke out on the frontier of the North West Province. As a regimental doctor assigned to the government of Madras, Ross was ordered to proceed directly from Secunderabad to Bombay to await further orders.[117] Coming so soon after an important breakthrough, this disruption seemed cruel and unusual. Not only were clinical cases and mosquitoes unavailable there, but Ross simply did not know how long he would remain in this post. When he arrived in Bombay, he was relieved to learn that he had been posted to Kherwara, Rajputana, where he hoped he would receive a permanent post or resident surgeoncy.[118]

The appointment proved to be only temporary. Dreading Secunderabad, Ross inquired, lobbied, and pleaded with Indian authorities about obtaining the post of Madras bacteriologist D. D. Cunningham, securing a resident surgeoncy in Rewa, being attached to a projected Health Institute supported by Indian princes, or being transferred to Bangalore. As his requests were denied, rejected, or ignored, Ross became more desperate and more demanding. He urged Manson to lobby the Indian secretary of state for a special malaria commission.[119] "I don't mean to say that the Government of India will not do their best; but they have so many claims upon them that without urging and reminding they are, I feel, very likely to forget our humble investigation. They are also apt, I fear, to forget that their humble servants have exigencies as well as themselves and that sometimes they cannot be kept waiting for ever." Ross warned, "Unless [the Secretary of State] acts, the investigation will be almost certainly deferred until the plague ceases — a poor prospect, because the plague will probably last for years yet. By that time I fear that, unless something unforeseen happens, my services will no longer be available." [120]

Manson consulted with Crosthwaite and Joseph Fayrer, the former president of the India Office Medical Board (1874–95). Both discouraged him from contacting either the secretary of state or the viceroy. Circumventing the government of India would "set the backs of the Indian officials up and do no good." For his part, Fayrer recommended a private word with James Leslie Cleghorn, director-general of the Indian Medical Service (1895–97). Manson reported to Ross that if Cleghorn was to be influenced by public pressure, the article in the *British Medical Journal* should have a positive effect. "The notes by Thin, Bland-Sutton and myself appended to your article will show Cleghorn what people think of you." [121]

Beyond waiting to hear from Cleghorn, Manson tried to humor Ross. He stressed how Ross would improve his prospects by advancing the theory. "I feel that if you chucked it now you would regret the step ever afterwards for some one else would enter in and reap the harvest you have prepared with so much labour. If you succeed in proving the mosquito theory and if then the Indian Government will do nothing for you such a howl will go up from this side that they will shake in their shoes and have to mend their ways sharp." In any case, there was always America. "If still they refuse you then apply to the home government and if they refuse there is America which won't." [122]

In late January 1898, Ross finally received a special appointment for malaria research. He acknowledged Manson's assistance and the importance of metropolitan publicity: "I fancy the sanction must have been obtained before, probably as a result of your and Dr. Thin's remarks in the *B.M.J.*" [123] This appointment was quite an improvement over his regimental position. Ross would work under the director-general for six months at 1,000 rupees per month, and would have access to the one laboratory maintained by the government of India. There was a catch, however. Ross had six months to complete his work on the mosquito-malaria theory and was expected to investigate the cause and transmission of kala-azar, a disease that was raging in Assam. [124]

Within days of arriving at the Calcutta laboratory, Ross immersed himself in work. [125] But malaria cases were difficult to come by, and mosquitoes were not consistently available. Nor did grey (or barrel-backed) or dapple-winged mosquitoes, which fed on infected blood, exhibit pigmented cells. These early difficulties set back the completion of the proof: "My failure to find pigmented cells in the mosquitoes referred to is annoying as it pushes back indefinitely our prospects of obtaining complete proof shortly." [126] The difficulty of securing an adequate supply of research materials induced Ross to work analogously on sporozoa infecting birds, *Halteridium* and *Proteosoma*. [127]

This decision was a practical one, but was also strategically important. Beyond their convenience as experimental subjects, an important advance in avian sporozoa research had just been made in the United States; this would later shape Ross's understanding of the *plasmodium*. In February 1898, Manson informed Ross of a discovery by William MacCallum. MacCallum had shown that the pigmented cells, or zygotes, of *Halteridium* were in fact the offspring of sexual forms, that is, flagella and pigmented spheres. [128] "You should go over MacCallum's observations on halteridium and see if it is correct. If the polymitus is a fertilising factor in the halteridium cycle then the flagellated body of malaria is also a fertilising factor in the plasmodium cycle. And if this is the case, and the fertilised crescent-derived sphere becomes transmuted into a travelling-cell-piercing vermicule in the stomach of the mosquito we have the explanation of the pigment in your mosquito stomach cells; they are carried into the cell by the vermicule." [129]

Through a process of elimination, Ross produced pigmented cells in grey mosquitos that fed on birds infected with the *Proteosoma*. He fed ten grey mosquitoes on *P. reliticum*-infected larks and sparrows. In five out of nine, he detected pigment, either in the cellular form or in clumps. Ross also noticed sig-

nificant growth in pigmented cells in sacs that protruded from the wall of the
stomach lining into the body cavity.

> I find that [they] exist constantly in three out of four mosquitoes fed on proteosoma and
> increase regularly in size from about 4μ after about 30 hours to about 40μ after about
> 85 hours. . . . After about 49 hours many of the cells are found to be quite hyaline, that
> is free from vacuoles. After 72 hours almost all the cells look like spherical, almost clear
> bubbles and are easily seen by low power. The pigment appears to get less and less the
> older the cells are, until it is entirely absent sometimes after 72 hours. In most of the
> cells the pigment is contained in or upon a small internal sphere.[130]

On 21 March, Ross triumphantly wrote to Manson, "My wish is that you
were here to share with me the pleasure which I have experienced yesterday
and to-day in seeing your induction being verified. . . . I am producing pigmented
cells ad libitum by feeding grey mosquitoes on larks infected with proteosoma.
This, of course, means the solution of the malaria problem." Ross exaggerated
slightly. What he found proved that the pigmentation was the beginning of the
sexual cycle of the *plasmodium* in the mosquito. It certainly underscored the
vital relationship between the mosquito and the parasite. But Ross still had
to follow the development of the zygote and confirm the mode of transmission
before the theory was demonstrated.[131]

Manson was excited by Ross's latest letter. "I need not tell you how de-
lighted I was to hear of your success. Dawn seems to be near. It carried the
promise of a brilliant day. Depend upon it all your work will carry a rich reward to yourself and to mankind." But Manson urged caution in making the
announcement while assuring Ross of his credit. "Be very sure of your position; accumulate proofs; try for the human malaria mosquito. When the thing
is certain send it to me if you like and I will take care that it is properly recognised." This last promise partly reflected Manson's intention that the discovery
be firmly Ross's and secondarily British. He reminded Ross, "The Americans
will be working hard I have no doubt this summer and so too will the Italians
but I think you are well ahead of them all."[132]

Finding evidence of sporulation would virtually prove the original hypothesis. Ironically, Ross's failure would lead to a radical revision of Manson's hypothesis. Manson assumed that once the flagellum lodged in the cellular structure, the next stage of development involved the production of spores, which
would continue to develop in the mosquito even after its death. Ross under-
standably assumed that the sac would burst and fill the body cavity of the dead
mosquito with infective spores. To his surprise, Ross found little immediate evidence of sporulation: "I have kept dead mosquitoes until they have fallen to

bits—no development of the coccidia of 4th and 7th days. They resist longer in the stomach tissues, but evidently degenerate—capsule shrinks, contents contract and become yellow, & ultimately bacteria enter." [133]

Since Ross assumed that the developmental process continued in the mosquito, he inferred that the coccidia must burst in a living insect. The absence of spores and the presence of empty sacs fortified this inference. By examining the development of pigmented cells over several days, he noticed the sudden disappearance of pigmentation. During the next two weeks, Ross closely examined the contents of the sacs and their dispersal in the body cavity. He observed what appeared to be internal striations, which turned out to be germinal rods. At the time, Ross did not know what to make of the function of these rods. But on June 26 he found, in one six-day-old and one eight-day-old mosquito, rods that clearly burst out of their containing cells, lying among the scales and muscles of the thorax. Initially, Ross thought that they might have a reproductive function, but changed his mind. "The rods appear to be too numerous for this & sometimes *all* the coccidia in a mosquito are rod containing ones. They must evidently get into the insect's circulating fluid for some reason." [134]

Dissection enabled Ross to identify the destination of the rods. By dividing his mosquitoes between the thorax and abdomen, Ross initially found rods more numerous in the thorax cavity than in the abdomen. On occasion, rods were more numerous in the head than in the thorax. By chance, Ross noticed that "a delicate structure dropped out of the cervical aperture" when he was separating the head from the thorax. "I noticed at once that the rods were swarming here and were even *pouring out* from somewhere in streams. Suddenly to my amazement, it was seen that many of the cells of this *gland contained the germinal rods of protoeosoma-coccidia within them*." Further inspection revealed a lobe saturated with the rods, which poured out just as they had from the original coccidia when it had been opened. [135]

The lobe aroused Ross's curiosity. Once he had opened the delicate head, he found not only the gland but also a duct "*which led straight into the structures somewhere between the eyes*." Again, the cells were saturated with rods. Subsequent dissection convinced Ross that the duct led to the "head piece, probably the mouth. In other words it is a thousand to one, it is the *salivary glands*." Ross elaborated on the relationship of the rods to the salivary ducts:

In all probability it is these glands which secrete the stinging fluid which the mosquito injects into the bite. The germinal rods, lying, as they do, in the secreting cells of the gland, pass into the duct when these cells begin to perform their function, and are thus poured out in vast numbers under the skin of the man or bird. Arrived there, numbers of them are probably swept away by the circulation of the blood, in which they immediately begin to develop into malaria parasites, thus completing the cycle.[136]

Before Ross could be certain, he intended to infect a healthy bird. On 25 June 1898, he took three healthy sparrows that had been found to be free of parasites. On that evening and the evenings that followed, he subjected the sparrow to the blood meals of a mosquito that had fed on infected sparrows on 21 and 22 June. Ross found that "all three birds, perfectly healthy a fortnight ago, were now simply swarming with proteosoma, twenty parasites & more in one oil-immersion." Ross reached similar results when setting infected mosquitoes on healthy sparrows and baia: "Both had proteosoma, the sparrow a few, the baia fairly numerous." Ross concluded, "I think that I may now say Q.E.D., and congratulate you on the mosquito theory indeed. The door is unlocked, and I am walking in and collecting the treasures." [137]

No Vindication: Manson, the Revised Theory, and the British Medical Association

The timing of Ross's infection experiments with sparrows could not have been better. In the fall of 1897, the Council of the British Medical Association invited Manson to preside at the newly established tropical disease section at its upcoming annual meeting in Edinburgh in July 1898.[138] Once Ross had reported, in March, evidence of intercellular pigmentation in mosquitos that fed on sparrows infected with proteosoma, Manson requested slide preparations for presentation at the Edinburgh meeting. "I am looking forward to receiving the specimens. I hope to receive them in time for the British Medical Association Meeting in July. Their exhibition will be in itself sufficient justification for the institution of the Tropical Section at their annual meetings." [139]

Even though the stakes appeared higher than ever, Ross's ability to continue to work on the theory became more uncertain. His special duty appointment was to expire in August, and he was also expected to submit his report on *proteosoma* in May and then concentrate on kala-azar.[140] There was hardly any time to return to *plasmodium* without an extension of his appointment. Further, the publicity surrounding the mosquito-malaria relationship generated interest and attracted competitors. By the late spring and early summer of 1898, Giovanni Battista Grassi, Italy's foremost zoologist, and Robert Koch, Germany's leading bacteriologist, had channeled their energies into the elaboration of the sexual cycle of the *plasmodium* as well as the identity of the specific species of mosquito.[141]

In this context, Manson harnessed the one resource he knew how to exploit: metropolitan publicity. By mobilizing support for Ross's work, Manson attempted to secure not only more time for Ross to complete his research but also the priority of discovery of the mosquito-malaria relationship. On this occasion, the coordination between Manson and Ross was flawless. In March, Ross forwarded slide preparations to Manson and other investigators in Europe; these arrived in late April.[142] Shortly after Ross submitted his report, "Cultivation of Proteosoma, Labbe, in Grey Mosquitoes," in late May, Manson published an abstract in the *British Medical Journal* based on Ross's letters.[143]

Leaving little to doubt, Manson unilaterally declared the theory proved in Ross's name. "Indeed, [Ross] is now thoroughly convinced that the mosquito-malaria theory is sound, and that he proved it."[144] He also made use of the testimonials of Laveran and George H. F. Nuttal, formerly associate in hygiene at Johns Hopkins University.[145] Neither went so far as Manson, but their eminence as international authorities undoubtedly lent credibility to Ross's work and, by extension, to the theory itself. Nuttal wrote, "I have seen the preparations referred to by Dr. Manson in the foregoing article, and consider that they bear out the interpretation put upon them. It is very important that these most suggestive and valuable observations should be followed up, and every encouragement given to such original investigations." Manson translated Laveran's letter: "It is probable that it will now be easy to find the excorporeal form (*la forme de resistance*) of the parasites in external media. The discovery of Dr. Ross appears to me as to you, to be of very great importance. It is a great step forward in the study of the evolution of the haematozoon of birds, and very probably also in that of the haematozoon of malaria. I have shown the preparations to M. [Élie] Metchnikoff, who shares my opinion."[146]

Manson used this occasion not only to "place on record Ross's claims to priority" but also to settle some old scores, specifically "to vindicate [himself] from the charge of unscientific and unwarrantable speculation." Even though the original theory was based on circumstantial reasoning, he felt particularly ill used by his critics. "I have been stigmatized as a sort of pathological Jules Verne, and hinted at as being governed by 'speculative considerations,' and as being 'guided by the divining rod of preconceived idea.' "[147] With the demonstration seemingly near at hand, Manson defended his public style of scientific investigation with aplomb. "Work undertaken with the object of advancing knowledge is most economically expended if directed by 'speculative consideration' and 'preconceived idea,' provided these considerations and ideas are founded

on facts, and compatible with ascertained facts." In any case, Ross had verified the hypothesis. "The speculation in question has certainly guided Ross to
further and important facts, all of which point to the conclusion I venture to
indicate."[148]

For Manson, Ross's work was as much about the vindication of British
science as it was about his integrity as a man of science. In an editorial in
the *British Medical Journal*, Manson pleaded for continued support for Ross.
"Surgeon-Major Ronald Ross's most recent work on the mosquito in malaria
. . . shows that in this particular line of investigation for once our countrymen have been observing, reasoning, and proving, whilst their Continental *con-
frères* were still only speculating." In the same breath in which Manson congratulated Indian authorities on Ross's appointment, he insisted that they had
a moral obligation to do more: "Surgeon-Major Ross has opened a vast new field
for further work, and we do not doubt that if he be assisted and encouraged, his
labours will result, sooner or later, in not only a great increase of knowledge,
but in great benefits to a huge suffering humanity. The Indian Government must
not stop here. It is its manifest duty not only to retain him in his present work,
but to provide him with every assistance he may require."[149] Ironically, Ross received a further six months' extension of special duty, but to work on kala-azar
in Assam.[150]

By late June, Manson had begun detailing plans for exhibiting the mosquito-malaria relationship at the BMA meeting. In a letter to Ross, he promised to make "a good show of the slides and shall take care to have the matter
well ventilated."[151] Through an elaborate display of slide preparations, photo-
graphs, and magic lantern projections of the development of the *proteosoma-
coccidia*, Manson hoped to carry all but the most confirmed skeptics. To this
end, he sought confirmation of sporulation. "I am anxiously awaiting your next
letters for I would like to be able to say at the B.M.A. meeting that the early
stage and the sporulating stage of proteosoma in mosquito had been found."
Consistent with his original theory, the next stage of the investigation involved
tracing the assimilation of spores into a number of generations of mosquitoes
and the transmission of the infective form into birds. "Then found, what next?
I suppose following the spore into other mosquitoes and into birds. This will be
delicate work and difficult but to you not impossible. This worked out you will
be able to tackle human malaria."[152]

Rather than confirming sporulation, on July 4 Ross's curiosity led him to
follow the germinal rods of the *proteosoma* into the salivary glands of the mosquito. The notoriously slow Indian mail kept Manson in the dark about the
revision in the theory until days before the Edinburgh meeting.[153] This delay

actually worked to Manson's advantage in mobilizing support for his theory. Without it, the discovery of transmission in the bite of the mosquito would have superseded, if not altogether discredited, the original theory, thereby making the extension of Ross's special appointment unnecessary. As it was, the promise of discovery was seductive. Based on Ross's report and slide preparations, Lord Lister, the president of the Royal Society, lent his support in a letter, which Manson duly forwarded to Surgeon-General R. Harvey, director-general of the Indian Medical Service. Manson also planned to spur the India Office to act out of institutional self-interest by proposing that the Colonial Office—where he had served as medical adviser since July 1897—attach two men from the Colonial Medical Service to assist Ross in the elaboration of the theory of the human *plasmodium*. "I mean to try for this. It will do no harm to ask; on the contrary it will show him that your work is appreciated at home." [154]

As the BMA meeting fast approached, Manson grew anxious; his state was not helped by a debilitating bout of gout.[155] Ross had not replied to his letters since early July. Manson was especially concerned about his report to the tropical disease section: Confirmation about sporulation was uppermost in his mind.[156] It would seal the theory and also justify his rather partisan statements in his 18 June abstract. More practically, official protocol prevented Manson from basing his report on Ross's official report until after he received sanction from Surgeon-General Harvey or after its publication. Neither occurred by 15 July.[157]

In the intervening two weeks, Manson stopped promoting his original theory and became a publicist for Ross's discovery of the role of the mosquito as the transmitter of the parasite to humans. With few days to spare before the Edinburgh meeting, Ross's letters and telegrams finally arrived.[158] The timing could not have been better: The Council of the British Medical Association asked him to give a demonstration of the malaria parasite before a combined meeting of the tropical disease section.[159] No one but Manson knew about Ross's latest discovery. In his presentation, Manson framed the reception of Ross's work in two related ways: he narrated the process of induction that had led to the mosquito-malaria theory, and he exhibited slide preparations that presented a narrative of a biological or sexual process in the mosquito, that is, the production of zygotes from the conjugation of crescents and flagella.

Manson saved the best for last: the announcement of the discovery of transmission. To be sure, the suddenness of Ross's discovery, some six weeks after the *proteosoma* cultivation experiments, was bound to generate a stir. But Manson added even more drama to the occasion by reading a telegram from Ross regarding his latest infection experiments. Dr. T. Edmonston Charles reported to Ross that the communication "created a furore." Some twenty years after the fact, William J. Simpson recalled the "profound sensation produced among members when Sir Patrick Manson read out a telegram . . . describing success in conveying Malaria from bird to bird by means of 'grey' mosquitoes fed on Malaria infected birds."[160]

*   *   *

The discovery of the transmission of the malaria parasite in the bite of the mosquito reveals the cultural politics involved in the production of knowledge about the empire. As a medium of imperial science, the Victorian medical press played a vital role in this process. Manson harnessed metropolitan publicity both to transcend the constraints of geography and to create an audience for the mosquito-malaria theory. But Manson did more than simply publish his theory. Over a four-year period, he systematically framed the suggestive research findings of Ronald Ross as British science. This appeal to the nation enhanced the cultural power of Ross's research in two related ways: It politicized the mosquito-malaria relationship as a source of national pride while expanding the cultural bounds of British science to include the empire.

Customarily, historians of tropical medicine portray the discovery of the transmission of the malaria parasite as a critical turning point for British medicine and colonialism.[161] The prospect of controlling the scourge of the tropical empire spurred new imperial initiatives such as the domestication of tropical medicine. But the establishment of the London School of Tropical Medicine in 1898 polarized relations between the Colonial Office and the medical profession. The new school, which Manson proposed as medical adviser to the Colonial Office, brought to a head nearly a half century of tension between the medical profession and the imperial state over the social production of imperial doctors. As I will show in the next chapter, the problem of tropical disease was as much about the control over the labor of doctors as it was about disease in the empire.

5
Domesticating Tropical Medicine
The Formation of the London School
of Tropical Medicine

I N the late 1890s, the British medical profession and the Colonial Office engaged in a heated dispute over the training of prospective imperial doctors. The designation of the London School of Tropical Medicine as a single portal institution for entry into the colonial medical services of the dependent empire ignited this dispute (Figure 14). As proposed by Patrick Manson in 1897, the London School trained prospective colonial medical officers as well as civilian practitioners who contemplated practicing in the tropical empire. But the privileged function of the school provoked protest from the profession at large. Some objected to the arbitrary decision process in selecting the Royal Albert Docks Branch Hospital of the Seamen's Hospital Society. Others, such as administrators of medical schools, resented the subordination of their courses to those of the new school. Still others regarded the whole affair as betraying a complete disregard for the authority of the profession to determine how best to train imperial doctors.

In light of the long-term involvement of the British medical profession in the processes of imperialism, it would be easy to view this dispute as an exception in an otherwise harmonious relationship with the imperial state. In truth, this conflict over tropical medicine reflected the historically uneven power relationship between the imperial state and the medical profession. The component parts of the imperial state, that is, the Colonial Office and the colonial governments, used their economic power over medical professionals to secure the cost-efficient delivery of health care to a highly decentralized empire. The Colonial Office recruited prospective imperial doctors from a large pool of underemployed general practitioners in the metropole; colonial governments deployed them in their respective colonial medical services. As employers, colonial authorities possessed a wide range of tools to maximize the labor and performance of imperial doctors as primary-care givers, ranging from discretionary salary increases and performance-based financial incentives to punitive checks on private practice.

The medical profession could not afford to ignore the economic exploitation of its brethren in the empire. For a profession unable to monopolize the provision of health care, the condition of imperial doctors mirrored the uneven power relationship between providers and consumers in a highly competitive domestic medical market. If anything, overcrowding in the profession during the 1880s and 1890s only strengthened the interest of all practitioners in defending the social position of professionals as salaried employees of the state. This social crisis spurred practitioners to seek out appointments in the colonial medical services as occupational safe havens. It also had the effect of broadening the call for professionalizing the colonial services, as the leverage of the

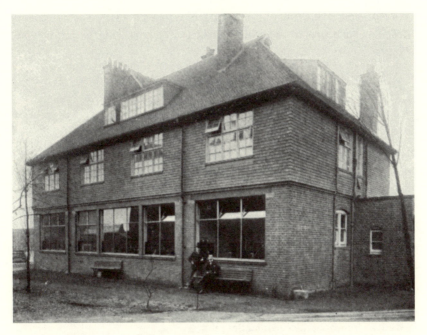

14. London School of Tropical Medicine, 1899. From Philip H. Manson-Bahr and A. Alcock, *The Life and Work of Sir Patrick Manson* (London: Cassell, 1927).

imperial state grew even more powerful. In a word, the profession wanted entry and career advancement in the services based on the specialist understanding of tropical disease rather than on the discretionary power of imperial and colonial officials as employers.

Furthermore, the shift in imperial policy toward the empire only intensified the domestic politics of tropical medicine. Colonial Secretary Joseph Chamberlain linked the long-term security of Britain to the economic development of its dependent empire, long known as the "white man's grave." Imperial officials were not wholly indifferent to the profession's call for special training in tropical medicine; they simply appropriated it on their own terms. Mandatory instruction in tropical medicine for prospective imperial doctors was designed not to enhance their social position but, rather, to maximize their labor as primary-care givers. This outlook reflected the long-term power of the imperial state as an employer of underemployed practitioners and the underlying political nature of the challenge of disease in the empire: how best to address the health concerns in a decentralized empire without micromanaging the delivery of medicine in the periphery. As this chapter will show, the establishment of the London School of Tropical Medicine proved to be a highly controversial solution.

The Politics of Tropical Medicine:
The Colonial Office and the Medical Profession

Customarily, the Colonial Office delegated health matters to the colonies. It nevertheless played an essential role as the chief recruiter of general practitioners for the local colonial medical services. With patronage control over some three hundred positions, the Colonial Secretary emerged as one of the largest employers of full-time civilian medical professionals by the end of the century. This leverage enabled the Colonial Office to secure the services of practitioners on its own terms. At most, it expected applicants to be between twenty-three and thirty years of age, preferably to be single, and to possess two qualifications (medical and surgical). Beyond these formal requirements, the applicants had to pass a health assessment and submit to an interview with a private secretary of the Colonial Secretary.[1]

These modest requirements did more than simply ensure the largest pool of potential applicants: They provided maximum flexibility in meeting the personnel needs of the empire (see Table 1). Forecasting vacancies was virtually impossible for a dependent empire whose staffing heterogeneity was matched only by its geographical diversity. Nor were imperial officials, who were ever conscious of economy, prepared to be burdened with a large supply of underemployed imperial doctors, as was the case in the state services or the Army Medical Department, the Indian Medical Service, and the Naval Medical Service. Instead, the Colonial Office staggered the appointment process to accommodate the personnel needs and fiscal imperatives of the empire. Prospective candidates submitted their applications in April. Those who were approved were then placed on the Secretary of State's appointment list. From this list, candidates were matched as vacancies opened during the year. Placement on the list did not guarantee an appointment, however. "No promise is given that any appointment will be eventually made," prospective applicants were warned, "and it is not possible to forecast either the number or the nature of the vacancies which will arise in the course of any given year."[2]

The Colonial Office could rely on this Dickensian appointment system because of the large pool of underemployed practitioners in Britain. Medicine was a popular calling; the profession could not assimilate all its members do-

TABLE 1   Appointments in the Colonial Medical Services of the Dependent Empire

Colony	Positions
British Guiana	45
Jamaica	56
Trinidad and Tobago	32
Windward Islands	22
Leeward Islands	25
British Honduras	5
Fiji	8
Sierra Leone	3
Gambia	2
Gold Coast	19
Lagos	5 (excludes 2 native appointments)
Ceylon	74 (excludes 8 native appointments)
Straits Settlements	11
Hong Kong	5
Gibraltar	2
Cyprus	3
St. Helena	1
Falkland Islands	2
Total	320

Source: "Medical Appointments in the Colonies," British Medical Journal, 28 August 1897, 558–59.

mestically. As Anne Digby has shown, the size of the fee-paying medical market was simply too small.[3] The existence of health-care alternatives, including home remedies, charitable medicine, low-priced medical dispensaries, and group contract services, made it hard for most practitioners to make a living. It is for this reason that those doctors who could not expect a viable career at home turned to the empire as a last hope. Some emigrated to establish practices in the fast-growing colonies of white settlement; others joined the state services. The modest entry requirements, together with the promise of a regular salary, made colonial service a tolerable career choice for those medical men who failed to succeed at home and/or were unwilling to make the long-term commitment that the state services required.

Moreover, the duties of imperial doctors did not require specialized training. Many availed themselves of the growing number of medical reference books on disease and illness in the tropics, or "warm climates," which were undoubtedly geared to practitioners in the metropole who contemplated practice in the empire.[4] Imperial doctors thought of themselves chiefly as primary-care givers who were expected to serve the health-care needs of European personnel and

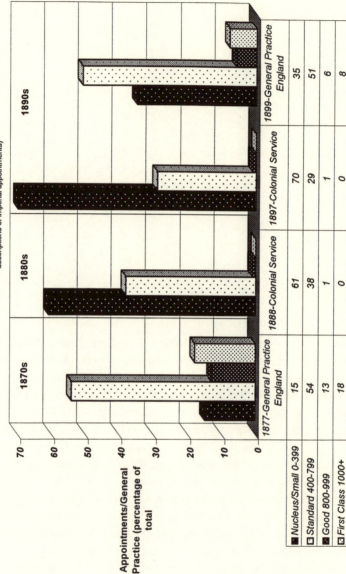

(Data derived from percentages based on samples of advertised positions in Britain and published descriptions of imperial appointments)

Appointments/General Practice (percentage of total)

	1877-General Practice England	1888-Colonial Service	1897-Colonial Service	1899-General Practice England
■ Nucleus/Small 0-399	15	61	70	35
▣ Standard 400-799	54	38	29	51
▦ Good 800-999	13	1	1	6
▨ First Class 1000+	18	0	0	8

Salaries/Net Income (pounds sterling)

*Salary Information for Britain is based on the study of salaries by Anne Digby in *Making a Medical Living* (Cambridge: Cambridge University Press, 1994)

15. Salaries for general practice in Britain and imperial appointments in the dependent empire.

their families and colonial charges as resources permitted. Most appointments involved taking charge of a medical and/or sanitary district, which could be quite extensive. Within these districts, officers attended the local hospital or poorhouse, oversaw sanitation, and/or performed vaccinations.[5]

Once a practitioner had accepted an appointment, he quickly became the financial captive of the colonial service. Even before being dispatched to a colony, imperial doctors were expected to purchase costly outfits, including clothing, camp cutlery, and a medical kit, as well as medical guides.[6] Base salaries varied from colony to colony, but they were low compared with average salaries at home (see Figure 15).[7] Salaries ranged between £100 to £300 for probationers and some district medical officers and colonial surgeons, between £400 and £700 for most district officers, and up to £800 for the chief medical officer of the Gold Coast colony.[8] To be sure, housing and travel supplements diminished the high cost of living in the empire. However, imperial doctors still lost ground, because salary increases were not automatic. They were awarded at the discretion of the colonial administrator or governor after the completion of a probationary period—lasting from two to three years—or after a fixed number of years of service, and were capped at a maximum salary level.[9]

While private practice was one of the attractions of imperial appointments, it was a privilege that colonial governments controlled. As a rule, newly appointed colonial surgeons were prohibited from engaging in private practice. (This was the case in Jamaica, Trinidad, British Guiana, and Hong Kong.) Where private practice was granted, it was generally used as an inducement for district officers with otherwise meager base salaries in Trinidad and Tobago, the Windward Islands, the Leeward Islands, Cyprus, St. Helena, the Falkland Islands, Fiji, and Gibraltar. Even when private practice was granted, officers were advised not to subordinate their official duties to private gain. In Ceylon, private practice was reserved for subordinate officers, "who are mainly recruited from among gentlemen born in the island but possessing British diplomas. In British Guiana, district officers who held additional public posts for stipends, such as charge of the Public Hospital in Georgetown or the Lunatic Asylum in Berbice, were barred from private practice. Besides these restrictions, the threat of disqualification for a coveted pension discouraged imperial doctors from pursuing private practice. (European personnel in West Africa were excepted from this provision.)[10]

Colonial governments used other incentives to maximize the labor of imperial doctors. In the Leeward Islands and British Honduras, for example, medical personnel received fees for *successful* vaccinations, postmortem examinations, courtroom appearances, and executing lunacy and burial certificates. In Fiji, they received capitation fees for treating indentured laborers. Stipends were awarded to medical personnel for assuming additional duties, such as taking charge of public institutions, for example, the civil prison or the lunatic asylum in Gibraltar; or serving as the officer of health in Lagos; or acting as ex-officio inspector or resident surgeon of the Lock Hospital, superintendent of the civil medical hospital, or health inspector of emigrants in Hong Kong.[11]

Practitioners were well aware of the prospects for a career in the empire. Queries about colonial appointments and their replies, carried in the medical press, reflect the career uncertainty of doctors in Britain and the frustration of imperial doctors. "West Indian," writing to the *British Medical Journal*, asked about appointments in British Guiana. "Are they worth applying for? Are they desirable appointments for a married man with a wife and family to accept?" [12] "X, Y, Z" provided the following facts for consideration:

The salary ranges from £200 to £300 a year, or thereabouts, and is, I believe, stationary. Private practice is sometimes, but not invariably, allowed. Movement from place to place is not infrequent. Absence from home for days together on tours of inspection is often requisite in large districts. House rent is high, and accommodation often very inferior. Servants require high wages, and are very independent. Houses are dear and inferior as a rule, except in Jamaica, and one or more houses are usually requisite for the work of the appointment. Carriages are dear and inferior, and one is almost a necessity where there is a lady. The cost of passage out is very heavy.[13]

W. Munro, formerly of St. Kitts, warned: "On the whole, I should not advise a married man with a family to go out to a West India colony, unless for some definite reason." [14]

Other correspondents alerted intending candidates to misleading local announcements for medical appointments. "M.D.," writing from the Central Province of Ceylon, regarded the advertised "emoluments" in the *Ceylon Observer* as only a "pleasant fiction." "The salary here is not really the money paid to a common clerk or storekeeper out here, and is barely sufficient to provide for the necessaries of life in the Coffee Districts, where a rupee has not the purchasing power of a shilling in England, and where the requirements are more." [15] Another "M.D.," who forwarded an editorial in the *Ceylon Times* announcing the salary reduction for imperial doctors by estate owners, warned "young medical men to think well before coming out here." [16]

Practitioners in Britain and in the periphery were sensitive to other labor practices that diluted the status of being a registered medical professional. Writing from Grenada, a "Registered Practitioner" viewed the appointment of unregistered practitioners to government positions as the unintentional consequence of a "misapplied regulation" that required "striking off of names of practitioners for change of address without giving [a change of] address."[17] But "Another Registered Practitioner" was far less charitable: "It may interest your correspondent to know that not only are many senior practitioners who are not on the Register employed by the Colonial Office, but that many junior practitioners have lately been appointed whose names are not on the Register, and, further, that several Colonial medical appointments have of late years been conferred on medical men not possessing a registrable qualification."[18] "A Member B.M.A.," who reported that unregistered doctors were employed in British Guiana, complained, "The laws affecting the medical profession are surely intended to protect its members; but, as administered, it would appear that its orthodox members are the only ones subject to the 'pains and penalties.'"[19]

The medical press did more than simply open its correspondence pages to practitioners in the empire; it also took a partisan stance by rising to the defense of imperial doctors. As a result, the press transformed the experiences of practitioners dispersed throughout the empire into a direct challenge to the economic and social interests of the profession at home. Greater than the fear of death was the "bugbear of the service" in British Guiana and Demerara, the *Lancet* declared. The fact that nearly half of the medical personnel were dismissed or resigned confirmed a local report that "the cause of drain on the service was not only inadequate remuneration, but the harsh and unworthy conduct of superior officials."[20] An editorial two months later warned colonial authorities of dire consequences if the condition of the service did not improve:

While the service is in its present disorganised state, we cannot recommend anyone who values his independence of action, or has any wish to uphold the dignity of his profession, to enter this colonial service. A "strike" of candidates is probably the only form of pressure that will tell upon the authorities, who, by their indifference to the complaints and representations of those who have entered the service, seem to show that, so long as there are men to fill the vacancies as they arise, they have no interest in the welfare of their servants.[21]

The conditions of service in British West Africa were little better. The *British Medical Journal* deplored the remuneration for imperial doctors. "What are the inducements offered? The highest rate of pay to which a colonial surgeon, in the worst climate in the world, can hope to attain, is £500 *per annum*; and before this salary is reached, six years of dreary service must be spent in the dismal region known as the 'white man's grave.'" In such a climate, the minimum age (fifty-five) and seven-year service requirement needed for a pension seemed to be little more than a cruel joke. "What the chances are of a man in such a climate surviving to enjoy a pension at the age of 55, is not a difficult calculation." The *British Medical Journal* also placed authorities on notice to reform or suffer the consequences:

We cannot promise colonial surgeons who have committed themselves to service in the West Coast of Africa that the Colonial Office will be induced by any representation of ours to do them tardy justice; but the voice of this Journal is far-reaching, and we can and do raise a note of warning to intending candidates for such employment. We can do something to "stop the supplies"; and the Colonial Office should be made aware that other taskmasters have been starved into compliance with the claims of right and justice.[22]

Even as the profession objected to the exploitation of imperial doctors, they asserted their cultural authority over the empire by appropriating the problem of disease, especially malaria. This metropolitan discourse on disease in the empire reflected the profession's entanglement in the cultural production of British imperialism. Malaria had long been viewed as a disease that originated in the environment, so medical writers ascribed the presence of malaria in the tropical world to the comparative failure of the indigenous societies to master the natural world. As a metaphor for backwardness, malaria framed Europeans in the tropical world as agents of civilization. Their death and debility symbolized the limits of civilization; hence the representation of the tropics as the "white man's grave." Conversely, the perceived immunity of the indigenous inhabitants to disease confirmed their backwardness while reinforcing the binary opposition between the healthy temperate world and the diseased tropical world.

By the 1880s, the meaning of malaria had changed. While malaria still signified the backwardness of indigenous societies, it ceased to bound the scope of European expansion. On the contrary, the acceptance of the *plasmodium* parasite now made the conquest of malaria no less than a test of national character (see Chapter 4). In announcing the formation of a malaria commission, a writer for the *Lancet* insisted on the need to ensure the spread of British civilization with as few deaths as possible. "What of the future? If our commerce, if our missionary enterprise, if our efforts at introducing the blessings of civilisation into the country are to be successful, it will apparently, as in other parts of the world, only be attained after the sacrifice of innumerable lives and at a great expenditure of money."[23]

The *British Medical Journal* decried the inadequate attention to tropical diseases in national terms: "It is not right that we should essay to govern millions of human beings, and withhold from them the full measure of civilisation;

TABLE 2   Growth of the Medical Profession in England and Wales, 1861–1901

Date	Numbers
1861	14,415
1871	14,692
1881	15,116
1891	19,037
1901	22,698

Source: Data complied from *Census Reports for England and Wales* for 1861, 1871, 1891, and 1904.

nor is it seemly that we in England should have to go for years to France and Germany for textbooks on a subject in which England should lead the way."[24] Six months after this diatribe, the *British Medical Journal* announced the creation of a lectureship in tropical diseases at St. George's Hospital, London. Manson's visibility as an authority on tropical disease, particularly on *filariasis*, secured him the post. Designed for medical graduates contemplating practice in East and South Asia and Africa, the course consisted of twenty lectures on selected diseases.[25] Other courses were subsequently established at other London medical schools, including Charing Cross Hospital, St. Mary's Hospital, Middlesex Hospital, and Westminister Hospital.[26]

Spurring metropolitan interest in tropical disease was social change within the profession. Between 1861 and 1881, the medical profession grew by only 5 percent.[27] This modest growth masked an impressive increase in the number of entrants to medical schools during the same period. Student entrants averaged 1,200 in the 1890s.[28] By the end of the century, the size of the profession registered the impact of student demand. In 1891 and 1901 the profession ballooned by 26 percent and 18 percent, respectively (see Table 2).

A number of forces spurred the expansion of the profession after midcentury. First, medicine had long been one of the most direct routes for upward mobility, particularly for Scottish, Irish, and English doctors of modest means. The relative social and economic accessibility of Scottish and, later, provincial institutions of higher education made university medical degrees more affordable than those from Oxford or Cambridge or London University. The reciprocity provisions of the 1858 Medical Act technically abolished the requirement of London or English qualifications as a condition of eligibility for public positions. As a result, career opportunities were widened for medical men who had obtained their training in Scotland, in Ireland, or in the provinces, though the preference for English or London qualifications remained in force at the leading hospitals throughout the century.

Second, the expansion of the Victorian state in public health and general health produced a growing demand for qualified medical professionals. Opportunities included positions on passenger and merchant vessels, jobs in factories and mines, the growing state medical services for the poor and prisoners, and the creation of positions for local medical officers in the burgeoning cities of Britain.[29] These positions, as well as others, mostly supplemented the incomes of private practitioners. Besides a regular income, poor law appointments, for example, provided a vehicle to enhance one's visibility while cultivating prospective clients among the local governing elite.[30]

Paradoxically, growth exacerbated the underemployment of practitioners and pushed many to secure appointments in the state and imperial services. During his valedictory address at the Army Medical School in Netley, Sir Dyce Duckworth said as much: "Our profession is, in fact, overstocked, and the strife to gain a living in it is very great. Competition is now so keen that some of our humbler brethren are compelled to undertake duties entailing anxiety and serious responsibility for the most miserable remuneration. In times of commercial depression young men are wont to resort to our profession, and so, of late, our ranks have been preternaturally filled."[31] Even the *Lancet*, no friend of the colonial medical services, conceded as much: "Though complaints are frequently published in the columns of the *Lancet* of the grievances of colonial surgeons, there always seems to be a sufficient supply of candidates for the comparatively small number of such appointments as happen to be vacant."[32]

This crisis of the profession renewed calls for diminishing the manifest leverage of the imperial state over medical professionals. "No one can to-day look out on the stormy sea of medical professional life without seeing how devoid of organisation it is, and how fierce and deadly is the struggle to exist within the profession. Such conditions are as bad for the people and the State as for the physician himself, and call urgently for redress," wrote George Evatt when proposing the professionalization of the colonial medical services. For Evatt, a staff member of the Army Medical Department, competition based on professional knowledge, rather than the discretionary power of imperial and colonial officials, provided the key to enhancing the social position of imperial doctors and to improving the efficiency of the colonial medical services. Using the model of the Army Medical Department, Evatt recommended replacing patronage with competitive examinations for appointments. The Colonial Office would subsidize successful candidates while they received instruction at Netley in tropical diseases and bacteriology. "Great advantages would result from this training, and an esprit de corps and feeling of comradeship be given to the service from such training. The want of such hygienic training must be a drawback to an official service largely engaged in preventing rather than curing disease." In place of a subjective process of promotion, Evatt proposed creating a uniform gradation of ranks. Career advancement, like entry, would be based on competitive examination. "No man need be promoted who does not pass a test, who has not gone through a post-graduate course. Medical men in the fierce competition of civil practice grade themselves at once by energy and efficiency, or by the want of both. In official services classification has to come by authority, and hence the need of tests as stimuli." [33]

Evatt's proposal elicited a mixed response in the British medical press. "A Colonial Medical Officer" concurred that the service needed to be professionalized. But his endorsement of competitive examinations was qualified. While they were useful for determining initial appointments based on tropical disease instruction at Netley or St. George's, he preferred that service and seniority be the basis of career advancement. This preference probably arose from a number of factors, including the self-image of many imperial doctors as primary-care givers, the opportunity costs involved in preparing and/or sitting for promotion examinations, and the inchoate nature of the specialty itself. Nevertheless, he appealed to the profession to support professionalization: "I am sure that both the service and Her Majesty's Colonies would largely benefit by some such organisation as the foregoing, and I would beg all Colonial medical officers, and especially those who happen to be home, to use all their influence in support of the organisation of the service, and I also hope, sir, that you will lend the powerful aid of the *British Medical Journal* to this end." [34]

C. H. Eyles, a colonial surgeon in British Honduras, was far less sanguine. Eyles viewed a unified service as not only costly but also "outside the field of practical politics." The very decentralized nature of the service posed an insurmountable obstacle to a centralized service: "Is it possible or likely that a number of isolated communities scattered throughout the world, and living under every conceivable diversity of conditions, would federate for the express purpose of establishing a highly centralised department?" Invoking John Simon's *English Sanitary Institutions*, Eyles added, "Unsuitable as this state of affairs would be in even the small and compact area of England, nothing but failure could result if it were imposed on the scattered communities represented by our Colonies." [35]

The perspectives of Evatt and Eyles reflect the social and political realities that defined the relationship between the medical profession and the imperial state. If anything, the late nineteenth-century policy of constructive imperialism, which called for the systematic development of the tropical empire, only intensified those realities. Even though imperial officials had a vested interest in promoting the understanding of disease in the empire, this does not mean that they were prepared to cede to the medical profession control over the social production of imperial doctors. Instead, over a four-year period, they arrived at a political solution, one that simultaneously capitalized on its role as employer of practitioners and accommodated the decentralized nature of the empire.

Institutionalizing Tropical Medicine:
The Formation of the London School of Tropical Medicine

One by-product of the metropolitan discourse on tropical disease was the growth in influence of the medical adviser to the Colonial Office.[36] Beginning in the 1870s, the Colonial Office retained practitioners in London, Edinburgh, and Dublin to assess the physical health and psychological fitness of prospective employees and imperial servants who sought medical leave or applied for their pension benefits. The narrow scope of these duties resulted from the practical needs of the imperial state as a metropolitan employer of civilians. Yet the 1890s generated a stream of unsolicited advice and products on the treatment of illness and the prevention of disease in the empire.[37] Lacking their own "in-house" expert, imperial officials turned to Dr. Charles Gage-Brown. Even though Gage-Brown provided advice as a courtesy, he was in a unique position to channel official interest in the problem of tropical disease. Indeed, the personal relationships that he developed among doctors in the empire, imperial officials, and members of the profession in London enabled him to operate as an influential conduit of information between the periphery and the metropole.

While on leave in London in the spring of 1895, John Farrell Easmon, chief medical officer of the Gold Coast colony, called on Gage-Brown. Easmon, who was the highest-ranking West African in the entire Colonial Medical Service at the time, lobbied Gage-Brown to support his proposed training program at Accra. Unsatisfied with the preparation of newly appointed doctors, Easmon attached such doctors to the colonial hospital at Accra for two months. During this period, he conducted a short course on the endemic diseases of the region as well as the local details of sanitation in and around Accra. With a large medical department of twenty-two doctors, dressers, and nurses, this practice enabled him to standardize the quality of health care while supplementing the knowledge of personnel.[38]

There was certainly an element of self-interest on Easmon's part in lobbying Gage-Brown. He tethered his proposal to a request for three additional assistant colonial surgeons. A staff of twenty-two proved inadequate for the department's basic needs. Substitutes for personnel who became ill were not available; the extension of public health and medical facilities in Accra as well as the provision of regular service at the outstations of the colony demanded additional personnel. Further, the prospect of a capitation fee for newly appointed imperial doctors was attractive to Easmon: It supplemented his salary as chief medical officer when colonial regulations prohibited private practice.[39]

Gage-Brown endorsed Easmon's proposal. It directly addressed the preparation of imperial doctors. "I fully believe that, if time can be made available to [Easmon], and to the Juniors, for lectures and clinical instruction by him a sound and systematic method of treatment can be learned. Then will be the best of teaching—bed-side instruction," Gage-Brown wrote to Chamberlain. Gage-Brown did more than simply endorse Easmon's proposa; he expanded it. "But there is the further question how it can be made available for those who are appointed to Sierra Leone, Lagos, the Niger Protectorate or any other stations." By broadening participation, Gage-Brown transformed a colonial responsibility into an imperial one by proposing instruction in Britain itself. "It was as comprehending the whole that I made my suggestion concerning Netley or a London Special course," he explained in a letter to Chamberlain.[40]

The fact that Gage-Brown's memorandum was forwarded to Chamberlain indicates the degree to which imperial officials were interested in addressing the training of prospective imperial doctors. Indeed, the Colonial Office asked Frederic Mitchell Hodgson, the acting governor of the Gold Coast, for additional details. Hodgson, who endorsed the expansion of Easmon's training program as a way to enhance the regional influence of Accra as well as raise revenue, doubted the suitability of courses in tropical medicine at Netley or at London hospitals. The lack of a regular supply of clinical material rendered these courses "more theoretical" than the one proposed by Easmon. But the availability of teaching material at Accra did not mean that special training was going to be inexpensive. In exchange for lodging, Hodgson estimated a £60 charge for each medical officer participating in the six-week training scheme. He also suggested that medical officers receive full remuneration during training and half pay while traveling to their designated colonies. Finally, Hodgson recommended that Easmon receive £20 per student for training each additional medical officer.[41]

As promising as the proposed West African training program appeared, its implementation proved to be practically and politically difficult. Comparing Easmon's £20 per student to medical instruction fees in London, Gage-Brown regarded it as generous to a fault.[42] For their part, imperial officials were anxious to secure a positive outcome before embarking on a novel initiative. Herbert Read, Chamberlain's private secretary, preferred soliciting the participation of other colonies only after success in the Niger Protectorate. Reginald Antrobus, however, feared a proprietary reaction from neighboring colonies, particularly Lagos. "Dr. Rowland will be sure to think (and he will probably be right) that he is at least as well able to train his assistants as Dr. Easmon; and in any case he would prefer to have his men on the spot ready for duty rather than train at Accra." [43] The Colonial Office grew increasingly uncertain about the likelihood of success of special training in the empire. Easmon's reluctance to accept less than £20 per student allowed it to drop the subject by early 1897. [44]

Although tabled, the subject of the training of prospective imperial doctors would engross imperial officials by the fall of that very year. Spurring this process along was Gage-Brown's successor as medical adviser, Patrick Manson. [45] Well before his appointment to the Colonial Office, Manson had been dissatisfied with the level of attention to disease in the empire in the metropolitan profession. Part of the rationale for establishing the Hong Kong Medical Society was to supplement the training of new arrivals to China. [46] Before the Hunterian Society in 1894, Manson chided the profession for its indifference. "England has willfully, or, rather, ignorantly and indifferently, shut her eyes to one of the biggest facts in pathology revealed during the present century. We seem to have gone to sleep where we ought to have been hard at work and in the foremost ranks of pioneers." [47] Shortly after securing his post, Manson intimated to Ross how he intended to make the most of his access to imperial officials. "It will bring many opportunities and if I can see my way I shall do my best to give a leg up to the teaching and study of tropical medicine. As things are, in this important section of medicine, are [sic] shameful. If I can get my way no man shall be able to get a license to practice tropical [medicine], at all events as a public servant." [48]

Three months after becoming medical adviser, Manson used a public occasion to mobilize interest in training prospective imperial doctors. The opening of the winter session at St. George's Hospital, where Manson had lectured on tropical disease since 1895, was largely a ceremonial affair. [49] But Manson undoubtedly understood that his introductory address would be widely reported in the medical and lay press. [50] In this address, he called for the domestication of the study of tropical disease in two critical ways. First, Manson recommended that medical schools establish an optional lecture course on tropical diseases and that licensing bodies, in turn, create a certificate in the subject. To make the certificate worthwhile to medical schools and students alike, Manson recommended that the Colonial Office give preference to those individuals who possessed such certificates when making appointments and require them for service in the tropical empire.[51]

Inside the Colonial Office, Manson's proposal for tropical medicine gathered momentum largely due to the efforts of Gage-Brown. Writing to Read, Gage-Brown reiterated the importance of special training for prospective medical officers by forwarding a copy of Manson's address. In a critical shift, Gage-Brown suggested special instruction in London, either in Manson's course at St. George's or at the Army Medical School, Netley, rather than in the periphery.[52] Administratively, London was more convenient for at least two reasons. Unlike Easmon's proposal, training in London offered no prospect of intercolonial competition or delay in the deployment of imperial doctors to their designated posts. Instead of complicating the role of the Colonial Office as a civilian employer, London-based instruction actually complemented it. As the national and imperial center of the profession, London functioned as a major recruiting hub for prospective imperial doctors.

Read followed up on Gage-Brown's suggestion and consulted with Manson. Concerned about the appearance of self-interest, Manson suggested exploring the possibility of attendance at the course at Netley.[53] Although Netley did provide instruction in tropical medicine, it was part of a six-month curriculum designed for the personnel needs of the Army Medical Department and the Indian Medical Service. Unlike these two services, the smaller, decentralized colonial services could not forecast the personnel needs of a far-flung dependent empire. Since the Colonial Office did not guarantee appointments to those on the appointment list, doctors were free to accept better situations. Though it was willing to make special provisions for imperial doctors, the War Office was loath to take spots from the army and Indian services. "Without knowing how many doctors you are proposing to send to Netley," wrote H. P. Harvey, private secretary to the Secretary of State for War, "and the period during which you want them to stay here, &c.—it is difficult for the Secretary of State to give formal assent to your proposal: we cannot tell if there will be sufficient accommodation available." [54]

This decision by the War Office created an opportunity for Manson. He proposed the establishment of a special school for prospective colonial medical personnel at the Royal Albert Docks Branch Hospital of the Seamen's Hospital Society.[55] The choice of the Albert Docks facility was no accident. Manson had served as consulting physician there since 1893. He was also well aware that the Society's management committee contemplated enlarging the hospital to accommodate the needs of the growing mainland population.[56]

In a matter of weeks, Read transformed Manson's proposed school into a single portal of entry into the Colonial Medical Service. Read did not draw up his plan from scratch but availed himself of the proposals that had been in circulation for several years. In stressing the advantages of centralized instruction to Charles Prescott Lucas—one of three undersecretaries of state of the Colonial Office—Read echoed Evatt and others. Prospective imperial doctors would be placed under the "formal supervision of our own Medical Adviser, who will be able to give us valuable information as to their capabilities, to see that the sort of instruction is given to them which is best suited to the various colonies to which they are sent, to keep closer touch with them in the Colonies as he will know them personally." He added that a special school would foster a distinctive service culture. "The fact that the Colonial Medical Service has a place of its own will promote spirit de corps [*sic*] and give it a better standing. If our men were sent (say) to Netley they would probably feel that they were only hangers on, and had no real connection with a place which is now on Army lines." [57]

As much as the proposed school provided an opportunity to shape an institutional identity for the Colonial Office, it still required significant administrative and financial resources. Obligatory instruction created the expectation of an appointment for those who completed the two-month course. But the Colonial Office had never guaranteed an appointment in the past, precisely because of the difficulty of forecasting the personnel needs of a highly diverse empire. To secure the willingness of candidates chosen from the appointment list to complete the course, Read proposed two departures from past practice. The first involved subsidizing candidates while they attended the prescribed course in exchange for a commitment to accept the first available vacancy. Read then dealt with the issue of appointments by recommending the consolidation of the colonial medical services of the West African colonies into one regional service. By a few penstrokes, the number of career posts in West Africa was increased to seventy-four. Adding these to temporary medical posts on railways, expeditions, and surveys, Read felt certain of an ample supply of positions for graduates of the school. If this experiment proved successful, Read suggested consolidating other services in the East and West Indies. [58]

Financing a school was another matter. The management committee of the Seamen's Hospital Society agreed to establishing the school, but opened up the course to other practitioners, undoubtedly to guarantee a regular source of operating revenue. In addition to increasing the number of beds from eighteen to forty-five, the renovated Albert Docks now would include a lecture hall, laboratory space, a library, and residential quarters. Of the estimated £13,000 in construction-related expenses, the Colonial Office was responsible for £3,500. [59]

Even though the Colonial Office technically administered a significant portion of the globe, it had no discretionary resources. With little choice, Read turned to the Treasury. Treasury officials viewed themselves as guardians of the interests of British taxpayers and were reluctant to approve nonbudgeted or extraordinary requests, particularly for the dependent empire.[60] In spite of Chamberlain's ambitions for the empire, they did not view grants or loans for unsecured projects as consistent with their public trust. Read requested a grant of at least half of the sum—£3,500—on behalf of exchequer-aided colonies whose officers were to be trained at the London School.[61] Although Sir Francis Mowatt, the permanent secretary, agreed, he stipulated that the "remaining moiety thereto be contributed by other Colonies and the Niger coast protectorate."[62]

This would not be the first time that Chamberlain had gone cap-in-hand to the Crown Colonies. On the strength of Ross's *proteosoma* cultivation experiments in India, Manson persuaded Chamberlain to lobby the Royal Society to conduct an investigation into the cause and transmission of malaria. A reluctant Royal Society agreed in the fall of 1898, but the cost to the Colonial Office was £5,000. Chamberlain hitched this request for the Royal Society malaria commission to one for £1,775 for the London School from the Crown Colonies. But the combined sum was not distributed equally among all the colonies. When asking Gambia, Sierra Leone, the Gold Coast, and Lagos for £3,500, he justified this request by insisting that these colonies were likely to benefit the most and that the exchequer-aided colonies simply were not in a position to contribute. Nor could Chamberlain ask the Treasury to contribute on behalf of the exchequer-aided colonies for the malaria investigation, because it had already contributed £1,775 toward the proposed school in their name.

Most colonies agreed to contribute.[63] From the perspective of colonial governments, these imperial initiatives possessed several advantages. Neither interfered with the day-to-day discharge of health care in the colonies. If anything, these initiatives complemented the primary-care orientation of the local medical services. Better-trained imperial doctors presumably would increase their efficiency, but this improvement would not necessarily translate into higher salaries. Most governments possessed neither the personnel nor the laboratory facilities to subsidize research into the causes of diseases, including malaria. Finally, the contributions requested were not recurrent drains on the colonial treasuries but onetime investments that promised long-term dividends.

While most colonial governments supported the initiatives, imperial doctors were less than enthusiastic. The very idea of special instruction in tropical diseases in London implicitly questioned their competence. In a resolution, government doctors in the Federated Malay States maintained that "it is rather advisable to establish schools for the study of tropical medicine in the tropics themselves where there are ready at hand abundance of material for clinical teaching, as well as experienced practitioners quite capable of giving the teaching required." Further, they objected to subsidizing metropolitan initiatives when opportunities for research were not encouraged locally: "As regards any contribution to be made to an external scheme for the promotion of the scientific research, the Congress was strongly of opinion that in view of the fact little or no encouragement is given by Government towards the promotion of similar objects locally that any money which might be considered available to spend in this direction should be devoted to similar purposes in the Federated States, where a much wider scope is offered for its profitable employment."[64]

A member of the elected legislature in Jamaica echoed the views of the Medical Congress's resolution. Dr. Johnston moved that the request for a contribution from the colony for the London School and the malaria commission be omitted from the budget. "The request for the money is an absurd one. Every part of the tropical world had its own peculiar diseases, and it was utterly impossible to train a medical man in England for service in Jamaica, India, or Africa. Why should a poor Colony like Jamaica be asked to give money to qualify for practice abroad?" Johnston preferred that the funds be used to improve hospitals locally in order to attract surgeons from England. "There were about 25 Jamaicans . . . in England and he would like to see the money spent on a new operating room made sufficiently commodious for the attendance of the young men coming out from England who could observe the diseases of the island as treated by qualified surgeons."[65]

The metropolitan profession felt particularly ill-used by the Colonial Office as well. While Read was negotiating with the Seamen's Society to use the Branch Hospital as a school, Chamberlain, in a circular to medical schools and licensing bodies, stressed the need for establishing lecture courses in tropical diseases. He was anxious to extend the "benefits of medical science to the natives of tropical colonies and protectorates, and to diminish the risk to the lives and health of those Europeans who, as Government officers or private employees, are called upon to serve in unhealthy climates." In order to make their duty their interest, Chamberlain held out the carrot of preference for applicants who attended such courses when compiling his appointment list:

So far, then, as this Department is concerned, Mr. Chamberlain would be glad if any scheme could be arranged by which an opportunity for special instruction in tropical disease could be offered to the student by the Medical Schools of this country, and would be prepared to support it by selecting preferably for Colonial medical appointments those candidates who could show that they had studied this branch of medicine, especially if some certificate or diploma to that effect were forthcoming.[66]

This circular omitted two important pieces of information, namely, that the secretary's preference was for placement on the appointment list and that those selected for appointments were required to complete the course at the proposed school before being dispatched to the empire. Until these details became public in November, the promised preference spurred medical schools to capitalize on a seemingly marketable course of lectures when the profession was in the throes of overcrowding. Medical schools as diverse as St. Mary's, St. George's, Charing Cross Hospital, University College (London), University College (Bristol), Durham University, Westminster Hospital, and the Royal College of Surgeons, Edinburgh, all replied that the subject was already receiving attention.[67] Others notified the Colonial Office of the imminent establishment of lecture courses. These included Middlesex Hospital, Victoria University, Liverpool, Yorkshire College, Leeds, Queen's College, Cork, and Queen's College, Belfast.[68]

Medical schools did not speak with a single voice, however. Several leading London hospitals were critical of, if not hostile to, Chamberlain's circular. The faculty at St. Thomas's Hospital did not believe that the subject was being neglected. George Rendle, secretary, reported: "They wish to point out that there are already four medical schools in London at which systematic instruction is given in tropical medicine, and that such instruction is open to all students and practitioners."[69] T. W. Shore, warden of Bartholomew's Hospital, volunteered that metropolitan instruction supplemented training "on the spot." "Good lectures, with cases in hand, in Bombay, Hong Kong, Singapore, Uganda, Sierra Leone, and George Town, Demerara, would be valuable to medical officers arriving in these localities, and might wisely be established, and attendance on them encouraged, or required, for the Colonial Medical Service. Such lectures, on the spot, would probably lead to real advances in the knowledge of tropical diseases and their treatment. Lectures in London would be interesting as reminiscences, and might, by establishing preconceived ideas of an obsolete type, do actual harm to the student when he arrives in the tropics."[70]

Still others regarded the incentive to create more courses in tropical disease as counterproductive. Guy's Hospital dean L. E. Shaw interpreted the colonial secretary's preference as a prerequisite for applying for colonial appointments. "We do not believe that any material advantage would accrue by adding to the number of the schools at which education is given, and are of opinion that any regulation, requiring a candidate to have attended a course of instruction in tropical medicine before applying for a Colonial medical appointment would diminish the number of suitable applicants without commensurate advantage." [71] Shaw was not alone; the replies from St. Thomas's, St. George's Hospital, and St. Bartholomew's used virtually identical language concerning preference.[72]

Even though this muted criticism was confined to official correspondence, the future site of the school became the focus of a bitter and public conflict between doctors of the Dreadnought parent hospital at Greenwich and the management committee of the Seamen's Hospital Society. In a letter to the London *Times*, Henry C. Burdett, a member of the management committee, appealed to the public for £10,000 for construction expenses and £3,000 in annual support. To underscore the commitment of the Seamen's Hospital Society, Burdett pointed out that "the teaching staff will consist of the senior medical staff of the Dreadnought Hospital at Greenwich, as well as the branch hospital, together with a number of teachers specially selected and attached to the new school." [73]

This seemingly innocent appeal was no such thing, according to three members of the Dreadnought senior medical staff. Senior Visiting Physicians Curnow and Anderson and Senior Surgeon Turner were not aware of the proposed school and had not authorized the committee to make such a public comment.[74] In demanding a public apology for this "discourtesy," the senior staff revisited an issue that had long been smoldering: control of the hospital. The medical profession had long resented lay control. While the money raised by lay governors helped to transform the Victorian hospital into a major site for surgical innovation and medical experimentation, lay control undermined the authority of practitioners as health-care experts and reminded them of their social subordination.[75]

To the Dreadnought senior medical staff, Manson was persona non grata: He appeared to serve the management committee to serve himself. Anderson and Turner had earlier complained that the committee should have consulted the senior staff before appointing a surgeon to the Branch Hospital.[76] Manson did not appear to mind, but after this dispute the visiting staff broke off communication with the Branch Hospital. Manson did not improve his standing by representing himself in medical directories as a member of the far larger and more prominent Dreadnought Hospital. After this episode, Manson stopped attending Society Staff meetings.[77] Nor did he help matters by illustrating the metropolitan profession's ignorance in tropical disease, in his St. George's address, by erroneously pointing to inaccurate inpatient diagnoses at the Dreadnought when they originated from the Branch Hospital.[78]

The politics of institutional control also extended to patients' bodies. One privilege that visiting staff received was the use of clinical cases for instructional purposes.[79] In exchange for a fee, medical students accompanied staff doctors on the ward rounds to observe diagnosis and treatment of clinical cases. Undoubtedly, the growing interest in tropical disease made the senior staff particularly attached to the teaching fees. They therefore worried that Manson and the management committee would collude to divert clinical cases from the larger parent hospital to the Branch Hospital.[80]

As the conflict between the senior staff and the management committee became more acrimonious, the Colonial Office announced its plans for instruction in tropical medicine for prospective colonial medical officers. Chamberlain's circular spelled out the relative roles of the London School and the British medical schools:

It is proposed that, as is at present the case, candidates for medical appointments in the British colonial possessions shall be fully qualified before they can be put upon the Secretary of State's list, that from this list a certain number shall be selected annually to fill the vacancies which may occur in the Colonial Medical Service, that the selected candidates shall be trained for a period of at least two months at the Seamen's Hospital, and that they shall then be sent to the colonies or protectorates to which they have been allotted. . . . In estimating the respective merits of candidates on the Secretary of State's list regard will be had to the fact whether or not they have already received instruction in tropical medicine.[81]

Once the privileged function of the London School became public, the bubble of interest that Chamberlain's circular had created among medical schools was deflated. If attendance at the London School was mandated, there was little incentive to establish lectures courses. "The success of this movement for affording instruction in tropical medicine in the Universities and the medical schools must depend largely on the recognition by the Govt [*sic*] of the University Certificate as evidence of proficiency," pleaded Andrew Davidson, a lecturer in tropical diseases at Edinburgh University and medical adviser for Scotland. Davidson appealed to Lucas to reconsider the subordination of all other tropical disease courses to those of the London School: "If, Sir, the very complete course—theoretical and practical—provided by the University of Edinburgh count for nothing, and if our students are compelled to go to London, there will be no inducement for students to attend the classes or work for the certificate; and this will strike a blow at the success of the movement." [82]

Ironically, because the Colonial Office had mobilized the interest in tropical medicine in the profession earlier, its announcement regarding the London School provoked a power struggle over the control of instruction. The power of the colonial secretary as employer was not in question, but the profession attempted to persuade Chamberlain to reverse himself based on the apparent flaws of the proposed site. "If compulsion is exercised on applicants for Colonial medical appointments, as seems to be implied in Mr. Chamberlain's letter, of course a regular supply of students will be at once forthcoming," the *Lancet* admitted, "but if there is no compulsion we question whether many will attend at such an inaccessible situation as the Albert Docks, and we doubt whether the variety of cases is sufficient to interest and instruct them for such a long period of three or four months." [83]

Several members of the Royal College of Physicians questioned the prudence of subsidizing an ill-chosen institution when Netley and a host of metropolitan hospitals could easily satisfy the needs of prospective imperial doctors.

Medical men connected with missionary societies and trading companies, along with those who in a private capacity propose to practice in the tropics, have open to them for the special study of these diseases the London and provincial schools of medicine where the subject is taught. Many of these are provided with bacteriological laboratories and all that is required for academic teaching. For clinical work the material afforded by the Dreadnought and its Branch . . . is available for those residing in London, while those resident in the provinces have valuable opportunities in this respect at such ports as Liverpool, Newcastle, Bristol, and other places.[84]

Edgar M. Crookshank, professor of bacteriology at King's College, offered a compromise plan. He envisioned a program of instruction in clinical and laboratory training in which students selected from a list of approved institutions. For clinical work, students enrolled at the London School—with the cooperation of metropolitan schools—would receive a ticket granting them "the privilege of being shown in the wards any cases of interest to colonial practitioners." Other students could attend a course of lectures either at the London School or at any recognized medical school. Both the lecture courses and the practical courses had to include a minimum six-week segment in a recognized bacteriological laboratory, completely equipped and fully staffed.[85]

Meanwhile, Manson's close association with the Branch Hospital and the Colonial Office provided an effective way to cast doubt on the process of selection of the future London School of Tropical Medicine. "Are we," sarcastically wrote the senior medical staff,

to understand that the offer of public money came from the Colonial Office solely to increase the accommodation of the hospital to which the medical adviser to the Colonial Office is attached, that the Committee deliberately kept their visiting officers of the Dreadnought in ignorance of their scheme until it had been decided to accept this offer, and to become responsible for the expenditure of public money. If so, was this done with only one possible teacher then at their disposal—the medical adviser to the Colonial Office himself?[86]

For William Broadbent, a leading member of the Royal College of Physicians, Manson's conduct had damaged the constructive participation of the College in the future school. "It is a matter of universal regret that anything should have arisen to interfere with the enthusiastic support [physicians] were disposed to accord. But, the College has taken the strong step of refusing to nominate a member to the committee." Broadbent even suggested that Manson defend his conduct before the governing body of the College. "I should think that Dr. Manson will feel bound, in the interests of the proposed institution, and as a matter concerning his personal honour, to appear at the next Comitia, and endeavour to remove the difficulties."[87]

The intensity of the controversy was beginning to wear on the nerves of imperial officials. A. E. Collins, private secretary to Chamberlain, ruled out offering Manson to the Comitia. "I would [give] no indication to the suggestion that Dr. Manson should appear before the College of Physicians. We cannot allow that distinguished body to settle our [affairs]." Instead, Collins thought a face-to-face conference of Chamberlain and Broadbent with Manson would defuse the dispute. "If Mr. Chamberlain could find the time to preside over this small conference, the explanation given in his presence would probably avoid the bad effect that will result from a conflict with the College of Physicians." Collins added, "We want public subscriptions and we cannot afford to disregard this annoying interference."[88] Lucas concurred, but snapped, "I really did not see what we have to do with family jams or what the College of Physicians or any other body has to do [with] the place which you select for a medical school, but I think with Mr. Collins that if you were to give Sir W. Broadbent and Dr. Manson an interview it would smoothe down matters."[89]

Even as the Colonial Office attempted to contain the controversy, matters grew worse. The publication of Broadbent's *Times* letter in the *British Medical Journal* scotched any meeting between Broadbent and Manson.[90] Nor did the attempts by the management committee to conciliate the senior staff by inviting their participation in the proposed school bear fruit: In April they resigned in protest.[91] But these gestures masked a far graver threat: the erosion of the proposed school as the single portal of entry to the Colonial Medical Service. Their worst fear came in the form of a request by Alfred Jones, the chief benefactor of the recently founded Liverpool School of Tropical Medicine, for recognition of its course in tropical medicine.

Jones could not be ignored. He was a vocal supporter of the empire, with extensive business interests in West Africa.[92] To the irritation of imperial officials, his concern for the empire extended to volunteering the advice of a homeopath in order to rid Africa of malaria.[93] However misguided, Jones was precisely the pro-empire type that was critical to the viability of Chamberlain's initiative on tropical medicine. In reply to Chamberlain's call for instruction in tropical diseases, Jones promised £350 for three years to develop a tropical disease research laboratory at the Royal Infirmary.[94] Although this donation would form the foundation of the Liverpool School of Tropical Medicine, Jones and members of the school committee sought more than a pat on the back. In a letter to Chamberlain, Jones requested not only a grant for the maintenance of the school and a donation for construction expenses but also recognition of the course as qualifying graduates for an appointment in the Colonial Medical Service.[95]

In a minute on Jones's requests, Lucas laid out the political problems of financial support and recognition of the Liverpool School. "But, if you make Liverpool a sister school, in the first place you water down your scheme at once, you have no longer one school, answering to Netley, for which you have secured a government grant and before it is opened, you have diverged into two: it may be a good thing but it is not the scheme which was put before the public. And accepted by them." Lucas doubted that the Colonial Office could seek further assistance from the Treasury without "any face." Second, there was every reason to expect that other institutions would seek recognition: "But if it is picked out from among the other hospitals to share with the Albert Docks Hospital the training of the selected, I cannot help thinking there may probably be an outcry, from King's College." Third, there was a real possibility that the Liverpool School, owing to its well-developed economic ties to Africa, might "attract more doctors for West African service than the London School." [96]

In denying the request for assistance, Chamberlain hoped that the matter of recognition for the Liverpool School would drop; it did not.[97] On behalf of the school committee, Jones asked if the Liverpool course could be substituted for the London School course.[98] The Colonial Office could not duck the question any longer. Lucas had little choice but to admit that the London School needed time before the Colonial Office could consider extending recognition to Liverpool. "All doctors appointed to the colonial service should before taking up their appointments be attached to the Albert Docks Hospital for at least two months. It is considered necessary to insist upon this condition until the proposed system is in full working order and has had a fair trial. Whether in the light of further experience the condition can with advantage be modified may be considered hereafter." [99]

This was hardly the beginning envisioned by Manson and the Colonial Office. Rather than inspiring the profession in the name of the empire, the London School of Tropical Medicine became a lightning rod of controversy. Even after the school opened, its long-term viability was clouded with uncertainty. To be sure, Chamberlain helped to retire the outstanding debt for enlarging the hospital facility by hosting a charitable dinner.[100] However, this generosity did not relieve the hand-to-mouth existence of the school. Nor did many members of the Colonial Medical Service avail themselves of private medical attendance at the Branch Hospital on a sliding scale.[101] As it turned out, student fees just covered operating expenses, in large measure because the teaching staff were only nominally compensated.[102]

* * *

Although medicine has often been seen as a "tool" of British imperialism, the relationship between the imperial state and the medical profession was not a harmonious one. The contentious founding of the London School of Tropical Medicine reflected the continuation of a long struggle over the control of the labor of medical professionals. Even though the members of the profession asserted their authority over the problem of tropical disease, the imperial state as employer determined the social conditions under which medicine was practiced in the empire. So, too, did the privileged function of the London School as a single portal of entry into the Colonial Medical Service reflect the power of the Colonial Office. If anything, the subordination of medical schools to the London School reflected the power of the imperial state to control both the labor and the social production of imperial doctors.

While the contentious founding of the London School revealed the social tension between the profession and the state, it also compromised the viability of the school as a research institution. Support from the British public was anemic, and student fees barely kept the doors open. Without an endowment, the London School could not pursue an independent research agenda, much less address the needs of the empire. It was at this time that Manson and the Colonial Office turned to the empire to subsidize research science in Britain. As the next chapter will show, the Tropical Diseases Research Fund reflected the historical social division of labor regarding the production of knowledge about the empire. Crown colonies complemented their primary-care orientation by supporting research careers and laboratories in scientific specialties, including helminthology, protozoology, parasitology, and entomology in Britain. This net transfer of resources from the empire to the metropole not only made possible research science at the London School and elsewhere but also laid the foundation for the hegemonic authority of metropolitan science over disease in the non-European world.

6

The Tropical Diseases Research Fund and Specialist Science at the London School of Tropical Medicine

T HE domestication of tropical disease research ignited another metropolitan conflict involving the imperial state and the London School of Tropical Medicine. Colonial Secretary Joseph Chamberlain hoped to promote research in disease and health in the empire domestically through the Tropical Diseases Research Fund. Although subsidized by Crown Colonies and the government of India, the Fund was only tangentially concerned with the explicit needs of the empire. Instead, as a new source of metropolitan funding, it rapidly emerged as an important institution in shaping the landscape of research science in Britain. This prospect, more than anything else, polarized the deliberations of the advisory board. The feuding between Patrick Manson and Sir Michael Foster over the location of specialty positions in protozoology and entomology revolved around the institutional politics of funding for metropolitan science. Ultimately, the London School prevailed, not because it was a more deserving institution, but because the Colonial Office had already designated it an imperial institution.

The politics of tropical research funding underscores the historically uneven power relationship between the imperial state and metropolitan science. Until the 1890s, the Colonial Office delegated the problem of disease to the colonies. The emphasis on primary care, together with medical crises, in the periphery created a space for the assertion of imperial leadership. Since the periphery had few institutional resources of its own, Chamberlain extended to the colonies a level of expertise that they were either unable or unwilling to provide for themselves by capitalizing on the dependence of the Royal Society on financial support from the imperial state. The later establishment of a regular source of revenue for imperial research enhanced the power of the Colonial Office. As this chapter will show, the Tropical Diseases Research Fund simultaneously consolidated the roles of the Colonial Office as an important source of expertise for the empire and as an influential patron of metropolitan science.

The Formation of the Tropical Diseases Research Fund

For most of the nineteenth century, Britain did not cultivate research into the diseases of its dependent empire as an official policy. Nor did the Colonial Office in London possess the personnel, much less the discretionary resources, to shoulder this responsibility. Its three medical advisers in London, Edinburgh, and Dublin mainly assessed the health of prospective and career imperial servants and did little else unless specifically requested.[1] As a department of state, the Colonial Office was entitled to the services of the medical officer of the Local

Government Board, whose salary it subsidized.[2] There is little evidence that the services of the medical officer were solicited, much less viewed as a resource for the empire.

This gap should be seen not as indifference or even as the perceived limitations of medical science but, rather, as a function of the social production of imperial medicine. As a large metropolitan employer, the Colonial Office recruited qualified general practitioners for the local medical services of the dependent empire. Nor did the imperial service attract specialists, much less researchers. On the contrary, imperial appointments were tolerable to underemployed general practitioners precisely because they did not require any further training beyond the minimum needed to be placed on the medical register. For colonial governments faced with limited human and other resources and potentially unlimited health-care demands, general practitioners proved to be highly functional. Beyond discharging their duties as primary-care givers at local hospitals, asylums, and prisons, imperial doctors also served in other capacities. Such a doctor might be the sanitary officer of a district, a public vaccinator, or a representative of the colonial government when giving testimony or certifying births and deaths.[3]

The very utility of general practitioners was not without its drawbacks. It circumscribed the authority of imperial doctors as agents of preventive medicine and virtually ruled out research as an integral component of their official duties. This did not mean that colonial governments were wholly indifferent to the health of the colonies or the colonized.[4] As a matter of fact, colonial governments authorized a wide spectrum of ordinances that dealt with general health. These covered financing public works projects such as establishing and maintaining water systems, improving the collection and removal of sewage, building hospitals and cemeteries, preventing the spread of rabies by regulating dog ownership, and imposing quarantine measures against cholera and plague.[5]

These and other measures depended not on the authority of imperial doctors but, rather, on a host of variables. These included the advice of sanitary engineers, previous encounters with infectious or contagious diseases, the commitment of the colonial governor or administrator, the availability of local financial resources, and the cooperation of property owners and other interest groups.[6] The very politically constructed nature of public health shaped the local response to the problem of disease. Predictably, neither imperial doctors nor colonial officials are at their best when faced with endemic or epidemic disease. Spasms of concentrated—and, not infrequently, counterproductive—activity punctuate long periods of seeming indifference.[7]

Imperial officials in London largely took little notice of infectious disease crises in the periphery. Even in the age of the telegraph, distance and economy conspired against ameliorative-action directives from the metropole. Yet by the 1890s, disease in the empire had begun to capture official attention. Spurring this shift was a twofold process. Unlike his predecessors, Joseph Chamberlain, as colonial secretary (1894–1902), called for a more active role for the imperial state in the administration of the dependent empire. Centralizing a highly decentralized empire, along the lines of the French model, was impractical. Chamberlain instead pursued his goal through imperial coordination. By taking the initiative in established arenas, such as the recruitment and training of imperial doctors, or reserach into disease which colonies were unwilling to do for themselves, Chamberlain made centralization politically possible.

Chamberlain's arrival at the Colonial Office coincided with a series of medical crises in strategically sensitive areas of Britain's African empire. Zululand, where tsetse fly disease surfaced in 1894, represented a critical region in the consolidation of British regional hegemony against the expansionistic Boer nation-state.[8] Uganda, the epicenter of the 1901 sleeping sickness epidemic, was no less important. This region not only formed the heart of the British East African Protectorate. It also insulated the higher reaches of Britain's most important trading conduit to the east—the Nile River Canal—from French and German encroachment.[9]

These crises provided Chamberlain with an opportunity to assert imperial leadership. Even though the Colonial Office lacked its own experts, Chamberlain was resourceful, even imaginative, in maximizing the relationship of the imperial state to the Royal Society. Despite its reputation for being a bastion of elite science, the Royal Society was not indifferent to support from the imperial state. This was especially the case because reformers within the Society sought to transform it from a "body of well-educated and cultivated men" into a "scientific institution of the highest rank."[10] With limited resources at its disposal, the Society in 1849–50 gladly accepted the Whig Ministry's support for science. Although the first government grant of £1,000 was little more than a gesture, the Society preferred to regard each annual renewal as evidence of a long-term commitment to science. At least this argument prevailed over a Treasury threat to terminate the grant in 1855.[11] Later, the Society's relationship with the state deepened through its supervision of the Science and Arts Department's Government Fund Committee (GFC). While the Society continued to receive its usual grant-in-aid, beginning in 1876 it participated in the disbursement of a further £4,000 annually for research. When the GFC was discontinued and merged with the Society's Government Grant Committee in 1881, the Society saw its annual subsidy balloon to £5,000.[12]

Roy MacLeod has shown that the government grant-in-aid to the Royal Society from 1849 to 1914 represented the single most important source of institutional support for Victorian and Edwardian research. During its sixty-year existence, this state subsidy, which totaled £179,000, subsidized some 938 individuals in 2,316 projects.[13] Although state support enabled reformers to transform the Society by promoting research among its fellows, this support did not come without strings attached. At the request of the Colonial Office, the Society organized a tsetse fly advisory committee to oversee the research of Surgeon-Major David Bruce.[14] Five years later, the Society studied malaria, again at the request of the Colonial Office.[15] In response to the epidemic visitation of sleeping sickness in the British East Africa Protectorate in 1901, the Society organized two research expeditions concerning the cause and transmission of the disease.[16]

In the short term, the collaboration with the Royal Society proved to be highly advantageous. The problem-orientation of these advisory/research committees enabled imperial officials to respond to uncertain epidemiological challenges with surprising flexibility. In an age of the mass press, the involvement of the leading scientific institution in Britain afforded welcome political cover: The Royal Society shifted attention from the Foreign and Colonial Offices to the investigation itself. This style of imperial science could not have been more economical. By utilizing personnel within the wider orbit of the imperial services and soliciting contributions from Crown Colonies as well as from the Royal Society, the costs associated with responding to acute medical and infectious disease crises were manageable.

At the request of the colonial governor of Natal and Zululand, Sir Walter Hely-Hutchinson, the army seconded Lt. Col. David Bruce, who was stationed in Pietermaritzberg, Natal, to work on the tsetse fly from 1894 to 1897.[17] Charles Wilberforce Daniels, a medical officer in British Guiana, received permission to represent the Colonial Medical Service on the 1898–99 malaria commission.[18] Several colonies subsidized the £400 salaries of Daniels's colleagues J. W. W. Stephens and S. R. Christophers for up to two years.[19] Herbert Read, Chamberlain's private secretary, charged the transportation and living expenses of the members of the sleeping sickness expedition to the budget of the Uganda Protectorate. The Royal Society, too, underwrote part of these initiatives from its annual subsidy. In 1896, the Council of the Society voted £200 for its tsetse fly advisory committee. It contributed another £600 toward the malaria commission in 1899 and was also responsible for the scientific outfit and "such *honoraria* for the expedition" for the sleeping sickness expeditions.[20]

Yet for all of its advantages, this style of research proved to be a mixed blessing. The very autonomy of the component parts of the research enterprise potentially threatened to undermine the whole apparatus. Bruce's unexpected recall to Pietermaritzburg interrupted his investigations into tsetse fly disease. Only after Governor Hely-Hutchinson secured a second leave could Bruce resume his work.[21] Even though the Royal Society was dependent on the imperial state, imperial officials could not take the Society for granted. Manson lobbied for the members of the malaria commission, including an entomologist, to assist Ross in elaborating the development of the parasite in the mosquito before proceeding to Africa to study blackwater fever.[22] Sir Michael Foster, secretary of the Society, stubbornly resisted harnessing the Society's credibility to the then-problematic mosquito-malaria theory.[23] In the end, a compromise was reached: Daniels visited Ross as an independent observer before rejoining the malaria commissioners in Africa.[24]

The problematic nature of collaborative imperial science spurred official efforts to institutionalize research science at the London School of Tropical Medicine. Unlike the Royal Society, the Colonial Office exerted direct influence over the school. Selected Crown Colonies had subsidized the establishment of the school; Read served on the management committee of the Seamen's Hospital Society, and Manson functioned in all but name as the official representative of the Colonial Office on the faculty. To be sure, in 1901 the course at the Liverpool School of Tropical Disease was placed on an equal footing with the London School course. But for all the above reasons, the London School was the preferred institution in the eyes of imperial officials.

As a matter of fact, Read and Manson had hoped that a generous British public would provide the necessary resources to institutionalize research science. But after the contentious founding of the school, appeals for an endowment failed to generate much, if any, public interest. At most, the gift of £300 for three years, from London merchant John Craggs in 1899, enabled the school to provide a traveling fellowship, for three years, to its most promising graduate.[25] Nor could the Seamen's Hospital Society apply to the Prince Edward Fund, a charitable foundation for hospitals, since the school's primary mission was educational.[26]

Whatever research activity the school engaged in usually mirrored Manson's scientific agenda. This reflected not only Manson's prominence but also his access to imperial officials, which opened up research opportunities that otherwise would have been beyond the means of the school. Once the Royal Society had confirmed the transmission of malaria in the bite of the mosquito, the Colonial Office, at Manson's request, authorized £500 for prophylaxis and infection demonstrations in the suburbs of Rome and in London, respectively.[27] The majority of the personnel engaged in these demonstrations were either

London School staff (Louis Sambon, instructor, and George Warren, laboratory assistant) or graduates of the London School (George Carmichael Low, Craggs Fellow) or related to Manson (that is, his son Patrick Thurburn).[28]

In 1901, the Colonial Office passed on to Manson a request from the Christmas Island Phosphate Company for assistance during an outbreak of beriberi among imported East and South Asian workers. Manson's son Patrick and H. E. Durham, a graduate of the Liverpool School of Tropical Diseases, participated in this privately funded research expedition.[29] Manson was also largely responsible for organizing the first sleeping sickness expedition, in 1900–1901, which included Low and Aldo Castellani, another graduate of the school.[30]

Clearly, the London School's limited resources restricted what it could practically do. It was for this reason that the three-month course stressed primary and preventive medicine, rather than training for prospective laboratory-based researchers. There were no scientific specialists on the staff, and there was only one general laboratory. Nevertheless, the teaching staff was eminently qualified for its teaching mission.[31] It was anchored by Manson, whose *Guide to Tropical Diseases* was the principal textbook; the other lecturers included Tanner Hewlett, Andrew Duncan, James Cantlie, Oswald Baker, William Simpson, Louis Sambon, Malcolm Morris, Treacher Collins, and D. C. Rees, the medical tutor, who would be replaced by Charles D. Wilberforce in 1901.[32]

The course itself was divided into two parts. The medical superintendent provided basic bacteriological and pathological instruction in the diagnosis, investigation, and treatment of disease. Clinical instruction in the wards and the outpatient department, provided by the staff attached to the branch hospital or to the parent hospital at Greenwich, represented the bulk of the course. Some eighty densely packed lectures on diseases and hygiene complemented the systematic and clinical portions of the course. In general, these lectures stressed practical knowledge about tropical diseases, namely, their geographical distribution, clinical history, and microscopic diagnosis and treatment, rather than providing specialized technological knowledge for future investigators.[33]

The final examination questions underscore the practical orientation of the course. Students were asked to describe the methods for demonstrating the Widal Reaction in typhoid and Mediterranean fever and for purifying water on the march; to distinguish between the *Anopheles* and the *Culex* mosquito and the different *filaria* embryos; to diagnose leprosy, syphilis, lupus, and malaria; and to describe the recommended treatments for cholera and Dhobi itch. The laboratory practicum tested for competence and little more. Students were asked to describe the steps to identify an unknown broth in a test tube, to stain blood samples for revealing the malarial parasite, and to identify abnormalities and determine the stage of infection based on microscopic specimens.[34]

TABLE 3   Enrollment at the London School of Tropical Medicine, 1900–1911

	First Session Jan.-April	Second Session May-July	Third Session Oct.-Dec.	Total for Year
1899	—	—	27	27
1900	24	27	23	74
1901	19	28	28	75
1902	27	31	33	91
1903	26	31	31	88
1904	37	41	37	115
1905	28	24	42	94
1906	21	32	42	95
1907	24	37	29	90
1908	30	37	45	112
1909	34	52	59	145
1910	40	53	44	137
1911	37	58	64	159
	347	451	504	1,302
		Total 1,302		

Source: *A Short Account of the Craggs Prize, 1899-1911*, pamphlet (London: London School of Tropical Medicine, 1912).

The emphasis on practical instruction did not check demand for the course. In fact, this emphasis, together with the privileged function of the course, represented its main attraction. For doctors contemplating practice in the empire or among the growing number of people in Britain who traveled or worked in the empire, research was the exception rather than the rule. During the first two complete years (1900–1902), enrollment consistently exceeded the twenty-student capacity for each of the three sessions (see Table 3).[35] Hoping to increase the number of students, school officials approved the renovation of the physical premises, which included remodeling the library and museum, expanding the laboratory space and lecture hall to accommodate up to forty students, and increasing the number of student living spaces from six to twelve.[36]

Operating revenue could only go so far in paying for the projected £9,000 renovation. Disappointed with the indifference of the British public, the school authorities as well as the Colonial Office looked to the empire for financial assistance. In 1902, the school dispatched Sir Francis Lovell, a former surgeon-general of Trinidad, to raise funds for the renovation project among colonial governments and wealthy colonial subjects; Lovell netted £3,000 in his first try. But a doubling of students required more personnel as well as more resources to place the school "on a broader and more permanent basis." Since the colonies had helped to subsidize the school and other imperial initiatives, Read turned to them again.[37]

In a memorandum on government support for the school, Read proposed inviting Crown Colonies to fund two traveling scholarships, increase the salary of the medical superintendent, and appoint an assistant superintendent as well as a curator of the museum and library.[38] But the colonies were not a rich uncle who could be tapped whenever the occasion demanded. Up to this point, Chamberlain had tied his requests to explicit practical goals, ranging from the understanding of the causes of malaria, tsetse fly, and sleeping sickness diseases to improved training for imperial doctors. Approaching colonies to commit scarce resources to subsidize the operations of a school in London, with no immediate benefit, ran the risk of discouraging, rather than encouraging, support in the empire. It was for this reason that Read's proposal underwent a major change before Chamberlain solicited Crown governors in May 1903.[39] Instead of linking contributions to the London School, Chamberlain proposed an even more ambitious scheme, namely, the creation of an imperial research fund. Although the scope and orientation of the proposed fund ruled out subsidizing the salaries of administrative personnel, it would provide resources for endowing positions in specialist science that otherwise would not have been forthcoming.

As it turned out, colonial governors were well disposed toward the idea of a centralized research fund: It would complement the mission of the colonial medical services. By stressing that priority would be given to the practical needs of contributing colonies, Chamberlain ensured that the funds would not be used for research that was not organized around solving a manifest public health problem. The existence of a centralized research body was also cost-effective: Large capital investments for laboratories and/or adding new personnel to the colonial establishment would be unnecessary. In a word, the proposed fund maximized the scarce resources of the dependent empire.

Imperial doctors were less than enthusiastic about the proposed fund. Some regarded centralized initiatives, particularly those that required local resources, as impractical. In stressing the local, the imperial doctors were being not simply provincial but political. The encouragement of research provided a vehicle to improve the health of the tropical colonies and the doctors' social position as colonial medical personnel. They wanted professional rather than menial careers; relief from routine duties and greater control over their time; and incentives to enhance their promise as investigators rather than degrade it. Dr. William Prout, colonial surgeon for Sierra Leone, said as much when he recommended the establishment of a regional laboratory in West Africa: "The difficulties in the past have been great. As a rule the staffs have been kept at their minimum working power, there is a great deal of routine official work, and medical officers, in other Colonies at any rate, have been liable at any moment to be moved from station to station." Prout added, "Nothing militates against accurate scientific observation as want of continuity, and if an officer, when he shows a special aptitude, could be detailed to scientific work, as was done some time ago by the Government of India in the case of Major Ross, I have no doubt valuable results would be obtained."[40]

Prout was encouraged by metropolitan initiatives, but they were no substitute for local research efforts. "A Commission [with] special qualifications and scientific training, such as has been appointed to visit the various Colonies, will no doubt do valuable work, but it must not be forgotten that the diseases which require investigation, such as so-called blackwater fever, cannot be made to order, and the trained observer who is always on the spot is more likely to have opportunities of research than those whose visits are only of a temporary nature." Nor were the tropical schools without their own critical deficiency: "Much is being done at home, at different places, notably London and Liverpool, to solve the problems of tropical disease, but these places must always suffer more or less from want of material." For Prout, these limitations, together with the manifest interest of the colonial secretary, persuaded him that the time had arrived for a local initiative. "I would suggest for His Excellency's consideration and that of the Secretary of State, whether the time has not come for the establishment on the West Coast of Africa of a thoroughly equipped laboratory for the study of tropical diseases."[41]

Prout's case was compelling. Even Foster and the acting colonial governor, Major Nathan, writing on behalf of the malaria commission, acknowledged the wisdom of encouraging research locally. In the final analysis, neither was able or prepared to do more than pay lip service to the idea. From Nathan's perspective, Sierra Leone was not in a position to subsidize a laboratory. "Without [private] assistance [from commercial concerns operating in the colony], or unless . . . an imperial grant is made towards it," Nathan wrote to Chamberlain, "I am doubtful whether the establishment of a fully equipped laboratory at Sierra Leone . . . would be possible."[42]

When responding to Chamberlain's circular regarding the Tropical Diseases Research Fund proposal, Charles Daniels, director of the Institute of Medical Research at Kuala Lumpur, reiterated the wisdom of promoting research in the periphery. Drawing on his experience as a medical officer in the British West Indies, Daniels found the official approach to tropical disease distressingly inadequate. Metropolitan-based scientific expeditions were not only rarely needed and costly but insulting to imperial doctors. "It is [not] encouraging to local men who are working on sound lines to have the fruits of their labours taken from them. The members of the C.M.S. by being treated in this manner are discouraged from the investigations of diseases, finding themselves placed in an inferior position."[43]

Daniels proposed creating a chain of regionally based colonial laboratories and a research track for promising officers. "Many difficulties would be avoided," Daniels confidently predicted, "if the authorities at the Colonial Office could see their way to the formation of a special Colonial or Imperial service for the work of such institutes." He added, "Such a service would be recruited from members of the Medical Services of the Colonies, directly from the Schools of Tropical Medicine or elsewhere, and members of the service might, if necessary, be lent to the teaching staff of a school, and paid by that school or employed in the rare cases where an expedition or commission was really required."[44]

Just as imperial doctors saw an opportunity to improve their social position through subsidized research, so, too, did the Royal Society. Sir Michael Foster chafed at the loss of autonomy in the Society's relationship with the imperial state. The provisional nature of the problem-based tropical disease initiatives was a source of frustration, largely because of the loss of control over the research agenda. Dependent on official initiative, the Society could only lurch from one new crisis to the next. Basic research into the properties and processes of causal agents gave way to isolating an unknown cause or, in the case of malaria, haggling over research priorities and/or personnel of the expedition itself. Further, the publicity surrounding these commissions placed the Royal Society under public scrutiny—something that it studiously avoided—when it did not fully control the research apparatus. In a word, the Society bore all the responsibilities of scientific research without any autonomy.[45]

Although frustrated by the nature of imperial science, Foster regarded official interest in science as an opportunity for metropolitan research science: Resources were limited. To be sure, science education after midcentury had begun to expand at the secondary-school level and, to a lesser extent, at the university level, but support for research in science as well as medicine remained modest at best.[46] As an entrepreneur of science who succeeded in consolidating research physiology at Cambridge University, Foster understood the particular financial challenges facing British research. As a leading scientist and member of Parliament for the University of London, he used his public visibility and private access to political elites to enhance support for science, particularly for institutions with which he was closely associated.[47]

Rather than simply accepting the uneven power relationship between the Society and the Colonial Office, Foster attempted to transform it by proposing the creation of a Royal Society tropical diseases research committee. Unlike past research committees, this one was to have a fair degree of autonomy. Its membership was weighted in favor of scientists: four, to two representatives from the Colonial Office. Instead of being dependent on medical crises or official initiative, the committee was to have the authority to establish and direct ad hoc research expeditions as well as the discretion to subsidize research at various metropolitan-based laboratories as it deemed necessary.[48]

In framing his proposal in a letter to Charles Prescott Lucas, one of three undersecretaries of state, Foster challenged the commitment of the Colonial Office to battling tropical disease: "The real question is [whether Chamberlain is] prepared to back a sustained attack against 'tropical diseases' . . . [or lead these] spasmodic efforts." The good intentions of the Colonial Office were both incomplete and costly.

The Malaria effort . . . is not complete, the Tsetse Fly business is not completed, in the sleeping sickness business time was lost before we could set to work, and the inquiry may have come to an end before the results are quite complete. Moreover ought we to wait for more or less a panic before we get stirred to undertake an inquiry? Ought we not to be always looking round, to see what needs looking into, and be prepared to look into it at once?[49]

Chamberlain was cool to the proposed role of the Royal Society. Besides complicating the financial assistance for the London School, Chamberlain regarded Foster's proposal as an attempt to shift authority on the question of tropical disease from the Colonial Office to the Royal Society. "[Foster] contemplates a prominent advisory board. I do not like this," Chamberlain informed Lucas after an interview with Foster.[50] As much as Chamberlain valued the assistance of the Royal Society, he was wary of relinquishing authority to scientists, particularly after Ronald Ross had embarrassed the Colonial Office by accusing imperial and colonial officials of placing economy above the health of personnel when promoting the application promise of the mosquito-malaria relationship. "It may become our Master and incur annoying expenses and take annoying precautions at the bidding of some enthusiast whose views may prove to be ephemeral."[51]

For his part, Chamberlain preferred an advisory board with only limited autonomy. The chief function of the board was to advise the Colonial Secretary on how best to allocate resources among existing institutions working toward the "improvement of life and health in malarious colonies." The composition

TABLE 4   Contributions of Crown Colonies to the Tropical Diseases Research Fund

Unit	Contribution (in pounds)	Years
Committed Support		
Imperial Treasury	500	5
Government of India	500	5
Malaria Commission Fund	180	one time only
Colonies		
Gold Coast	200	5
Southern Nigeria	200	5
Lagos	150	5
Ceylon	100	5
Straits Settlements	100	5
Federated States of Malay	100	5
Hong Kong	100	5
Trinidad	100	5
Mauritius	100	5
Fiji	100	5
Sierra Leone	100	5
Gambia	100	5
British Guiana	100	3
Grenada	50	5
Promised Support		
Basutoland	100	one time only
Orange River Colony	50	"
Malta	50	"
Seychelles	47	"
St. Kitts	25	"
Dominica	25	"
British Honduras	50	"

Sources: Enclosure in no. 3 Australia Mr. Lyttelton to Gov. G. R. Le Hunt, 31 August 1904, CO 885/9, 4–5, and "Sources of Promised Funds" table in minutes of first meeting of the advisory board, 1 November 1904, CO 885/9, 8.

of the board, not surprisingly, favored imperial control. Apart from one or two prominent London physicians, the medical adviser and representatives from the contributing Crown Colonies and the Colonial Office outnumbered the lone representative of the Royal Society.[52]

Foster's proposal never really had a chance. Once a sufficient number of colonial governors had agreed to contribute to the fund, it became moot (see table 4). Fourteen colonial governors committed nearly £1,500 annually for five years. Together with the annual contribution of £500 from the Imperial Treasury and the government of India, the dedicated income of the fund amounted to £2,500. The £312 promised by seven colonies, together with £180 from the Malaria Commission Fund, came to almost another £500 in onetime contributions.[53] Although Chamberlain did not remain in office long enough to see the Tropical Diseases Research Fund materialize, his successor, Secretary Alfred Lyttleton, brought it to fruition.[54] The short-term existence of the Fund—five years—together with the composition of the board, privileged the interests of the imperial state. At the first organizational meeting, the board's mission was made explicit: "In a word the main object of the Board is to secure the co-operation of the various agencies now or likely to be in existence for the improvement of health and sanitation in the tropical colonies and protectorates, and to ensure that full value is obtained for contributions which have been or shall be received." [55]

Considering the vast size of the dependent empire, £3,000 annually was a drop in the bucket. For research science in the metropole, however, the annual sum at the disposal of the advisory board was not an inconsiderable one. It was second only to the government subsidy to the Royal Society. More important, the Fund, unlike the Royal Society, subsidized institutions as distinct from independent investigators. This was an important distinction, insofar as resources for institutionalizing research science were scarce. The Fund, therefore, represented a powerful instrument in shaping the landscape of specialist science in Britain. It is precisely for this reason that the process of allocating imperial resources was such a politically controversial one. As the feuding between Manson and Foster will show, privileging the needs of the London School, as opposed to other metropolitan institutions, provoked conflict.

The Politics of Tropical Disease Research in London

Shortly after the establishment of the Tropical Diseases Research Fund, Manson lost little time in pressing the needs of the London School. At the first meeting of the advisory board, he requested a £1000 allocation for five years. These funds were intended to support salaries for positions in helminthology and protozoology and associated laboratory facilities.[56] Manson framed his application as a remedy to metropolitan indifference to core scientific specialities. "Apart from their special importance in the diseases of tropical and sub-tropical man, such studies and teaching should have a high economic value, for protozoology and helminthology are leading branches, and ought to be extensively taught as such, in veterinary medicine, more especially in colonial veterinary medicine." The indifference to these subjects compelled interested medical men to obtain their specialist knowledge either on the Continent or during scientific expeditions.[57] Neither approach allowed the systematic cultivation of the research resources of the empire.

Instead, Manson proposed to domesticate research by the addition of two research lectureships. After six months of study at the leading continental research laboratories, the two research lecturers would return to the London School "to take up research and a small amount of teaching." Appealing to national science, Manson was confident that such a course of action would wean Britain from its dependence on the Continent. "I believe such a scheme would add very greatly to our knowledge of the cause and prevention of tropical diseases of man and animals, and, moreover, turn out a number of highly qualified men, capable of advancing the subjects, and who would make the Empire independent of Continental experts, besides being of enormous assistance in helping the Colonies in the management of epizootics."[58]

Foster saw an opportunity in Manson's application for research science at the University of London. As Foster's clash with Manson over the mosquito-malaria theory indicates, he did not have an especially high opinion of Manson as an investigator. Nor was his opinion any higher of the London School and the other postgraduate institutions that began to proliferate in the waning decades of the nineteenth century. These institutions either provided remedial education, that is, instruction in subjects that the graduate "ought to have learnt before he was a graduate, but did not," or functioned as finishing schools, that is, as "a means of giving a polish to the student as he comes rough-hewn out of the examination, and so making him presentable." Perhaps the worst deficiency of postgraduate education was that it did not provide adequate scientific instruction or produce scientific knowledge. Predictably, Foster thought that the scarce resources of the Fund could be put to better use, namely, in the establishment of a dedicated research professorship in protozoology at the more prestigious University of London.[59]

In spite of his preference, Foster could not unilaterally insist that the position be located at the university without causing contention; it was the London School's application that was before the board. Instead, he used the opportunity to strip the school of control of the proposed positions. He recommended that the positions be provisionally located at the London School but that the Royal Society Tropical Diseases Committee approve the nominees for the two positions. Thereafter, Foster proposed that the London School become incorporated into the University of London. To make incorporation attractive to university authorities, Foster offered the protozoology and helminthology positions in lieu of an endowment.[60]

At first sight, Foster's reasoning for incorporation appeared compelling:

The London School was a weak institution. However, Foster's goal was not the well-being of the London School per se but, rather, control over a new research position. By proposing a joint position between the school and the university, Foster virtually asserted that no credible investigator would join the London School faculty. Nor did he make his proposal any more palatable by volunteering that the presence of a salaried instructor would cause discontent among the nominally remunerated lecturers at the London School.[61] Finally, Foster insinuated that the actions of the Seamen's Hospital Society were consistent with his own recommendation for incorporation. He reported that the Seamen's Hospital Society had sought affiliation with the university in February 1903. But, in an allusion to the school's precarious finances, he added that the application had stalled because the school had "no permanent endowment." [62]

The Seamen's Hospital Society (SHS) had pursued affiliation with the University of London, but not on the terms proposed by Foster. Established in 1829 as an examining body, the University of London had expanded its role to include teaching and research by providing two types of affiliation with external institutions. Institutional applicants seeking casual affiliation had to submit to an inspection by university officials to determine whether "the status of the school and qualifications of its professors are such as to render it worthy of affiliation." The second form of affiliation involved the incorporation of the teaching or research unit into the structure of the university. As this relationship was more lasting, applicants were expected to possess an endowment and to conform to university regulations concerning governance and the appointment of personnel.[63]

The SHS approached the University of London early in 1903, seeking simple recognition, not formal incorporation.[64] The Academic Council of the University authorized the SHS to request an inspection of the London School premises and evaluate its personnel. From the spring of 1903 until the early summer of 1904, however, the SHS did not request an inspection.[65] Its inaction was probably strategic rather than a clerical oversight. Even though the SHS sought only recognition, it is likely that the precarious financial condition of the school and the lack of salaried personnel made it uncertain about the outcome of its application. It was for this reason that Manson's application to the Tropical Diseases Research Fund was so important. In the event of a positive outcome, the SHS could at least point to the imminent addition of two funded positions and associated laboratory facilities. Moreover, support from the Fund could easily be invoked as evidence of the imperial, if not national, importance of the London School.

Before the board, Manson doubted that the type of person that Foster had in mind could be secured for £500. Manson also feared that a position held jointly with the University of London would mean losing control over the appointment, including the content of the course of protozoology and the division of duties between teaching and research. Such a scenario, he warned, "would remove control over him from the authorities of the School, and would perhaps be inconsistent with the constitution of the SHS, or otherwise found unacceptable to the Society."[66]

All members of the board, including Read and Lucas, thought affiliation was desirable. Affiliation would enhance the legitimacy of the school and possibly stimulate even greater student demand for its course and the study of tropical diseases more generally in the metropole. But the board could not reconcile the differences between Manson and Foster. It decided to defer a final decision about Foster's proposal until it could consult with Sir A. Rucker of London University and the Seamen's Hospital Society. In the meantime, Manson consolidated the position of the school. Before the first meeting of the advisory board meeting adjourned, he requested a £250 installment for "making preparations (equipment of laboratory, &c) for the establishment of a chair in protozoology." The board could not refuse, since the issue was not whether the London School should have the position or not but, rather, how it would be connected with London University. The board granted the installment.[67]

The Seamen's Hospital Society threw a wrench into Foster's strategy. It revived its application for simple recognition, then expressed to the board in no uncertain terms its preference for retaining control of the position. Tactically, SHS secretary P. Michelli stressed the London School as a teaching institution when communicating the SHS position. "It is felt that efficient teaching must be the best claim that such an educational centre as the London School of Tropical Medicine can have upon the Senate of the University of London; it is suggested that this can only be attained by all teachers in the school being under one definite administration so far as discipline and teaching are concerned." To this end, Michelli provided two possible scenarios regarding the appointment of the protozoologist. In neither case did the University usurp the authority of either the SHS or the London School: "(1) That the teacher in protozoology be nominated by the SHS, acting on the recommendation of the Committee of the LSTM, and subject to the approval of the Senate of the University of London; or (2) That in the event of the LSTM being admitted as a school of the University of London, the appointment of the teacher in protozoology be made by a joint Committee of the University and the LSTM."[68]

Ultimately, Manson prevailed. There was no need to be incorporated, since the University of London recognized the school and designated its course as one of six specialties that medical students could choose from.[69] Manson's proposal was cheaper. He proposed accommodating the two positions for £5,000 for a minimum of five years. This sum included salaries and laboratory setup. Even Foster conceded that the £500 salary was inadequate to attract an established research scientist.[70] While the Royal Society was prepared to increase the annual remuneration by an additional £250, the total estimated cost of endowing a research professorship at the university, including a laboratory with an assistant, was £30,000.[71]

In support of a motion to allocate the remaining £500 to the London School for the protozoology position for the year, Lucas explained the position of the Colonial Office: "The temporary character of any endowment from the Fund was a very great difficulty in the way of obtaining a competent man for the appointment; . . . the only solution of the difficulty appeared to be to accept Sir P. Manson's original proposal." But all was not lost for Foster. Lucas outlined the steps the Colonial Office had taken and intended to take to endow a research chair in protozoology at the University of London. "In view of the importance of the subject, there was no doubt room for both a teacher at the London School, as proposed by Sir P. Manson, and a university professor; and . . . Mr. Lyttleton had personally seen professor Ray Lankester and Sir Patrick Manson about the matter, and proposed, in the first instance, to ask the Rhodes Trustees for a grant of the requisite amount."[72]

Within a year of establishing the positions in protozoology and helminthology, Manson approached the board again. On this occasion, he requested funding for an entomologist. Mindful of the contentious nature of his first application, he began lobbying Read months before formally submitting his request.[73] This was particularly important, since the resources available to the Fund were limited and temporary. Donor colonies committed themselves to a five-year schedule of contributions, after which time the future of the Fund would be reviewed. Most, if not all, of the resources of the Fund were already committed among a range of metropolitan institutions such as the London and Liverpool schools and the Royal Society's Tropical Diseases Committee. Accordingly, any new request required either a deduction from the allocation to an existing institutional beneficiary or a corresponding addition to the Fund.

Manson turned to Read to find additional resources in the Colonial Office budget to fund the entomology position. In a note, he explained the need for an entomologist at the school: "Every month the importance of this form (insect) of agency is becoming more evident." Manson asserted that "a scientific study of the disease germ and the epidemiology of a disease conveyed by an insect is not complete or perhaps of practical value unless the entire problem is solved by a scientific study of the insect concerned." Appealing to Read's preference for economy, Manson limited his request to £300 for five years. Hedging, he also suggested a joint position with the Royal Veterinary Hospital, to whose students the London School had just agreed to open its course.[74]

Read was sympathetic to Manson's request. He found the requested amount modest and its purpose useful. In a minute on Manson's request, Read reported that there was a general consensus of expert opinion in support of the position. He noted that when Manson had referred to the subject at a student dinner at the London School of Tropical Medicine, Professor Blanchard, director of the Paris School of Tropical Medicine, had "warmly approved" it, as did the chief veterinary officer of the board of agriculture and Sir J. McFadyean, head of the Royal Veterinary College. Read was especially impressed by the support of Mr. Smith, the director of the agricultural department of the Transvaal in southern Africa, whom he described as "an eminently practical man." Smith believed that such a position would be most useful in filling positions in the future organization of the East African agricultural department.[75]

Once Read had received authorization, he cobbled together a funding proposal for the position in preparation for submission to the Treasury. What is striking, though not surprising, about Read's funding strategy for the position is that he placed the needs of the London School above those of the Colonial Medical Service. By replacing at least one principal medical officer position with a relatively junior medical officer position, Read projected a £200 savings; £150 was then to be dedicated to the entomology position for five years in the form of a Treasury grant. Read was quite confident that the Treasury would go along with his recommendation. He intended to show evidence of colonial self-help in promoting tropical disease research by recommending that Lagos, the Gold Coast, and Southern Nigeria be asked to contribute £75 annually for three years.[76]

With Read's support, Manson approached the board in November for £500 for five years for an entomology position at the London School. Foster endorsed the importance of an entomologist, but again was reluctant that the position should be located exclusively at the London School. Instead, he proposed that it be affiliated with institutions that he felt were more representative of research science, such as the University of London or the Lister Institute. Manson was adamant: The position must be located at the London School. He doubtless reminded the board that the authorities of the Seamen's Hospital Society preferred control over the position in the interest of its teaching program.[77]

Foster's reservations reflected not only his preference regarding the style of research to be supported but also the fact that the Royal Society stood to lose £500 for five years. The board had awarded the Royal Society's tropical diseases committee £500 annually for five years for ongoing sleeping sickness

research. To accommodate Foster, Read proposed asking the Treasury to add
£500 to the Uganda budgetary estimates for the Society, thereby "leaving the
£500 granted by the Advisory Board free." [78] In defusing a potentially contentious problem, Read further marginalized the Royal Society among the priorities of the Fund: It ceased being a recipient of imperial research funds. Once
the Treasury had given its approval, the board granted a £1,000 allocation to
the London School for the entomology position.[79]

*   *   *

The domestication of tropical disease research reveals that the power of
the imperial state in the metropole was integral to its authority in the periphery.
As in the case of the recruitment of prospective imperial doctors, the Colonial
Office used its leverage as a patron of metropolitan science to create a role for
itself in the empire as the source of scientific expertise. Through the Tropical
Diseases Research Fund, the Colonial Office subsidized careers in laboratory
science at the London School as well as at other metropolitan institutions. The
advisory board awarded the Liverpool School of Tropical Diseases an annual
grant of £500 for salaries beginning in 1905; another £500 increased this in
1907.[80] Cambridge University received £100 for a scholarship in medical entomology beginning in 1907 and another £100 in 1909 for expenses for the Quick
laboratory.[81]

These funding decisions served the goal of the imperial state: They maximized imperial resources for science while cultivating knowledge about disease in the empire. But it is important to recognize that these funding decisions
did not occur in a vacuum. No different from other forms of economic extraction that took place during Britain's imperial age, each allocation made by the
advisory board diverted scarce resources from the periphery to the metropole.
This diversion politicized tropical disease knowledge by institutionalizing an
unequal social division of labor between personnel in the metropole and in the
periphery. It diminished the resources available for fostering a culture of laboratory research in the empire and enmeshed metropolitan expertise in the subordination of imperial doctors as primary-care givers.

Retirement

At the age of sixty-eight, Manson resigned his position as medical adviser to
the Colonial Office. Since his return from China, Manson's health had steadily

declined. Prolonged bouts of gout left him bedridden for days. Arthritis limited his mobility to such an extent that Manson, who earlier had ridden the bus, was compelled to be driven to and from the London School at Albert and Victoria Docks. "I am afraid I am a permanent cripple and that [the] next attack of gout will floor me altogether," Manson confided to Herbert Read about his imminent resignation in February 1912. "In the public interest I should tender my resignation of the Medical Advisorship to the Colonial Office some time this year—certainly before the end of October. I feel I cannot face another winter in London." [82]

Apart from his poor health, Manson could survey his career with some satisfaction. Financially, he was in excellent shape. A regular supply of students, as well as medical practitioners headed for the tropical world, made his tropical diseases textbook a Bible of sorts and generated nearly £100 annually in royalty fees. But this source of revenue was a minor tributary compared with his main practice. Soon after being appointed medical adviser, Manson saw his modest £250–300 practice quickly jump to £1,000 annually. No doubt the publicity that he had generated for the mosquito-malaria hypothesis enhanced his visibility as a leading specialist in the metropole. At the height of his reputation, Manson generated between £4,000 and £5,000 annually.[83]

With these resources, Manson was able to place the family finances on a solid foundation. Henrietta and Patrick moved from their Queen Street townhouse to more comfortable rooms in Webeck Square. They also purchased a home and adjoining property in Lough Mask, County Galway, Ireland, which served as a retreat until they permanently relocated there. Here Manson recuperated from his periodic bouts of gout, pursued the only outdoor activity his fragile body could permit—fishing—and entertained friends and doted on his grandchildren.[84]

In addition to the financial security of his London career, Manson received a stream of honors for his work on behalf of the study of tropical diseases. Based on his involvement in the discovery of the transmission of the *plasmodium* parasite, the Royal Society elected him to the fellowship in 1900. The British Medical Association awarded him the Stewart Prize for the encouragement of the study of epidemic diseases a year later. He received the Fothergillian Medal from the Medical Society of London and the Bisset Hawkins Gold Medal for "advancing sanitary science" in 1905 from the Royal College of Physicians. In recognition of his service to the Colonial Office, he was appointed a Commander (in 1900) and a Knight (in 1903) of the Order of St. Michael and St. George.[85]

He was also regarded as a leader in the field at home and abroad. The

Society of Tropical Medicine elected him its first president in 1907. He gave
the prestigious Huxley Lecture in 1908. He received several honorary mem-
berships from the Manila Medical Society in 1903 and the Société de Medicine
de Gand and the Royal Academy of Turin in 1908. In 1904, the Cooper Medical School in San Francisco invited Manson to deliver the Lane Lectures. The
Tropical Medicine Society of the Republic of Cuba conferred on him the Socio
de Merio in 1908.[86]

For Manson, his greatest legacy was the London School of Tropical Medicine. To be sure, from a financial perspective the school was hardly out of the
woods. Lacking the security of an endowment, as late as 1910 the school existed
on a combination of student fees and general subscriptions.[87] Nonetheless, from
its modest beginnings at the branch hospital of the Seamen's Hospital Society,
the school had grown in more ways than one. By 1911, the original residential facilities, which originally had accommodated twenty, held thirty-eight; the
number of clinical beds had increased to fifty. In addition to a library and a
lecture hall, the school now boasted laboratory facilities for instruction and
research in protozoology and helminthology.

Epilogue
From White Man's Burden to
White Man's Grave

T WO years after Patrick Manson died in 1922, the Royal Society of Tropical Medicine and Hygiene established the Manson Memorial Medal (Figure 16). It was a tribute to his contributions to the field and to the Society. Since its inception, the Council of the Society has reserved the medal for distinguished workers in the field. In many ways, it serves as a suitable symbol for British tropical medicine. Its very name underscores the way disease in the tropical world has been and remains a product of European or Western perception. Symbolically, the Society's designation of the heirs to the father of the field connects investigators from the past, present, and future in a shared mission, namely, to protect the tropical zone from disease through Western medical science. If anything, the roll of medalists, who have been with few exceptions British, male, and white, has reinforced the normality of European authority over disease in the tropical world while simultaneously obscuring the legacy of imperialism in the making of British medicine and science.

As I have argued throughout this book, the history of tropical medicine is more than a story about disease in the tropical world. It reveals the critical role of imperialism in constituting British medicine and science in the nineteenth and twentieth centuries. The health care needs of the informal and formal British empire contributed to the growth, as well as the institutional development, of the profession at home. As part of the cultural production of imperialism, the representation of the tropics in the medical press as diseased or backward provided a space for constructing the image of Britain as an advanced and healthy society and British medicine as a tool of modernity.

British science participated in the imperial project as well. The high priority placed on the delivery of primary care in the dependent empire created a de facto social division of labor concerning the production of European knowledge about disease in the tropical periphery, whereby imperial doctors treated illness in the periphery and scientific specialists investigated their causes in the metropole. This division of labor created the conditions for the formation of the Tropical Diseases Research Fund. For twelve years, the Fund promoted the understanding of tropical disease by subsidizing specialized research careers and laboratories in Britain.

The involvement of metropolitan medicine and science in the imperial project in turn shaped the politics of tropical medicine in Britain throughout the twentieth century. As an extension of domestic institutions, the metropolitan study of tropical disease has long been justified by researchers and educators in paternalistic terms. The choice of the motto for the Royal Society of Tropical Medicine and Hygiene—*Zonae Torridae Tutamen*, or guardian of the torrid zone—was not surprising when the empire was at its zenith. The role of the

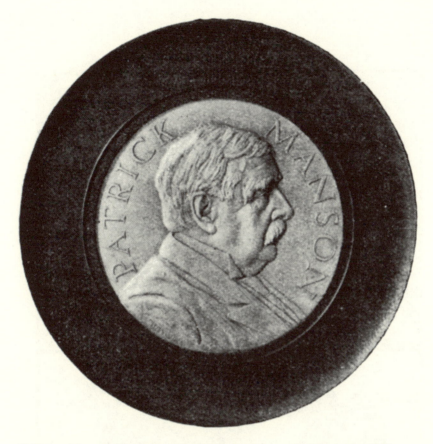

16. Manson Memorial Medal. From *British Medical Journal*, 22 September 1923.

specialist as guardian and the tropics as an object of danger paralleled Victorian tropes that justified the British imperial project in the name of the unique racial responsibility of white people—the white man's burden—and the threat that the tropics posed to the expansion of European civilization—the white man's grave.

The process of decolonization challenged the relationship of British medicine and science to the tropical world. Quite apart from shrinking the number of career opportunities for British practitioners, it also revealed the politically constructed nature of tropical medicine. Nonetheless, the leaders of the field have persisted in defending tropical medicine as if the empire still existed. In his 1961 presidential address to the Society, Sir George McRobert invoked cli-

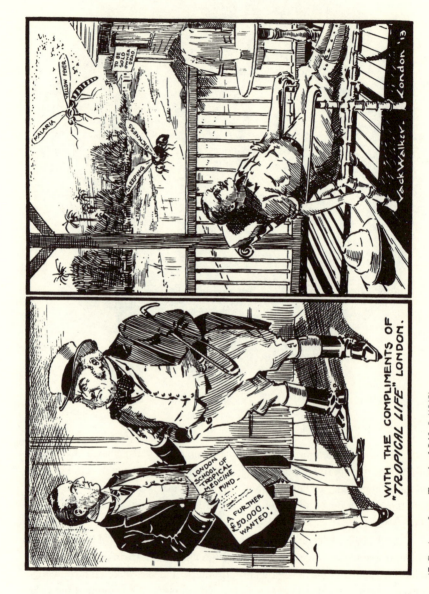

17. Cartoon from *Tropical Life* 9 (1913).

matic determinism when insisting on the spatial distribution of knowledge production between Great Britain and its former colonies. "Sir Andrew Balfour who did so much for tropical medicine used to refer to the benefit of a touch of snow on the mental powers. The highest grade of research work can be carried out only in invigorating climates: air-conditioning is not an adequate substitute." McRobert added that "two kinds of research workers are needed. High-power workers in temperate climates and well-trained competent workers for prolonged periods in the tropics. These men must have security of tenure and long-term prospects of employment guaranteed by a stable government. The former type should, however, visit the tropical scene of operations at intervals so as to keep in touch with actuality."[1]

Thirty years after McRobert's address, Kevin M. De Cock and three colleagues from the London School of Tropical Medicine openly questioned the relevance of the field in a letter to the *British Medical Journal*. "In summary, the urgent health problems of poor countries today are broader than those studied a century ago by Manson, the father of tropical medicine." By focusing on parasitic diseases, the field neglected the emerging infectious-disease crisis that accompanied urbanization as well as the health needs of millions of people displaced by natural disaster, war, and economic change. De Cock delivered the postmortem pointedly: "Tropical medicine would best be absorbed into the specialty of infectious diseases."[2] The *Lancet* was even more blunt: "It may be possible for the clinical services of tropical medicine to be absorbed into infectious diseases, but there is no reason for academic departments to be in London, or any other western city—rather, they should be where they belong, in the tropics themselves."[3]

Sir David J. Weatherall, a molecular biologist at Oxford University and 1998 Manson medalist, strongly disagreed with the *Lancet*'s stiff medicine: "Much of the critical work towards an understanding of the pathophysiology of common tropical infections, and research directed at vaccine production or treatment require advanced basic science technology," which, Weatherall volunteered, was available only in the developed world. "Surely the richer western countries owe it to the developing world to carry out research of this type."[4]

In case paternalism did not completely justify the need for the continuation of academic departments of tropical medicine, Weatherall deployed a related Victorian trope, a modified version of the white man's grave (Figure 17). By invoking the memory of Caroline Fraser, a Oxford University lecturer who died from malaria after failing to complete her regimen of antimalaria pills upon returning from a safari in South Africa, Weatherall framed the field as the barrier against external threats to the health and security of British society. "It is now a very small world and the tragic death of one of the brightest young academics in Oxford from cerebral malaria only a few weeks ago does not encourage the belief that 'tropical medicine' should be scrapped from the medical curriculum; if it 'moves to the tropics' who will remain to teach it?"[5] Ironically, if not perversely, shrinking resources and political support at the end of the twentieth century have forced the defenders of the field to embrace its past in order to secure its future in the twenty-first century. Manson would understand.

Notes

Introduction

1. Philip H. Manson-Bahr and A. Alcock, *The Life and Work of Sir Patrick Manson* (London: Cassell, 1927); Philip H. Manson-Bahr, *Patrick Manson: The Father of Tropical Medicine* (London: Thomas Nelson, 1962).

2. See Philip H. Manson-Bahr, *History of the School of Tropical Medicine, 1899–1949* (London: London School of Hygiene and Tropical Medicine, Memoir II: H. K. Lewis, 1956), 234.

3. By 1914 Manson's textbook *Tropical Diseases: A Manual of the Diseases of Warm Climates* (London: Cassell, 1898) had reached five editions. Manson asked Manson-Bahr to assume the editorship in 1919. "You might see the editor of Cassell's about a new edition of Tropical Diseases. This I would like you to bring out as Manson's Manual of Tropical Disease edited by Philip H. Bahr." See Manson to Manson-Bahr, 10 June 1919. Sir Patrick Manson Papers, Correspondence, F. 33, Wellcome Institute for the History of Medicine.

The investigation into the life history of the *filaria* worm represented a major area of research for Manson. Manson-Bahr's first monograph reflected this interest. See *Filariasis and Elephantiasis in Fiji; Being a Report to the London School of Tropical Medicine* (London: Witherby, 1912). For Manson-Bahr's marriage, see certificate in Sir Patrick Manson Papers, Folder 1 Personal and Biographical, box 25, Contemporary Medical Archives, Wellcome Institute for the History of Medicine.

4. Raphael Blanchard, a parasitologist at the University of Paris, first hailed Manson as "father" of tropical medicine at the presentation of a special medal to Manson at the 1913 International Congress of Medicine in London. See Manson-Bahr and Alcock, *Life and Work*, 226. On Manson-Bahr's efforts, see "The Dawn of Tropical Medicine, Being a Brief Account of the Life and Work of Sir Patrick Manson, 1844–1922," *Journal of Tropical Medicine* 34, no. 7 (1 April 1931): 93–97; "Centenary of the Birth of Patrick Manson," *Transactions of the Royal Society of Tropical Medicine and Hygiene* 38, no. 6 (July 1945): 401–417; and "Patrick Manson as a Parasitologist," *International Review of Tropical Medicine* 1 (1961): 77–129.

5. Manson-Bahr and Alcock uses the term "lad of parts" *Life and Work*, 2. See also Manson-Bahr, *Patrick Manson*, 3. For a sustained analysis of this national myth as it relates to education in Scotland, see R. D. Anderson, *Education and Opportunity in Victorian Scotland* (Oxford: Clarendon Press, 1983).

6. Manson-Bahr and Alcock, *Life and Work*, 5; Manson-Bahr, *Patrick Manson*, 5.

7. Manson-Bahr and Alcock, *Life and Work*, 8–23, 24–37; Manson-Bahr, *Patrick Manson*, 10, 12, and 14–15.

8. Manson-Bahr and Alcock, *Life and Work*, 90–103; Manson-Bahr, *Patrick Manson*, 48–57.

9. For example, see Manson-Bahr "The Dawn of Tropical Medicine"; Shelia Wilmot, ed., *Medical Entomology Centenary: Symposium Proceedings, Royal Society of Tropical Medicine* (London: Royal Society of Tropical Medicine, 1978), 7; Bruce F. Eldridge, "Memorial Lecture: Patrick Manson and the Discovery Age of Vector Biology," *Journal of the American Mosquito Control Association* 8, no. 1 (March 1992): 215–19; and L. G. Goh and K. H. Phua, " 'By Whose Efforts the Tropics Have Been Made Safe': The Work of Patrick Manson," *Asia Pacific Journal of Public Health* 1, no. 2 (1987): 84–90.

10. The term is from Charles Morrow Wilson, *Ambassadors in White: The Story of American Tropical Medicine* (New York: Henry Holt, 1942).

11. Manson-Bahr, *Patrick Manson*, 1–2.

12. I discuss this perspective in the epilogue.

13. See M. Jeanne Peterson, *The Medical Profession in Mid-Victorian London* (Berkeley: University of California Press, 1978); Irvine Loudon, *Medical Care and the General Practitioner, 1750-1850* (Oxford: Clarendon Press, 1986); Anne Digby, *Making a Medical Living: Doctors and Patients in the English Market for Medicine, 1720-1911* (Cambridge: Cambridge University Press, 1994); Peter Bartrip, *Mirror of Medicine: A History of the British Medical Journal, 1840-1990* (Oxford: Oxford University Press, 1990); and Peter Bartrip, *Themselves Writ Large: The British Medical Association, 1832-1966* (London: BMJ, 1996).

14. For recent representative works, see David Arnold, *Colonizing the Body* (Berkeley: University of California Press, 1993); Mark Harrison, *Public Health in British India: Anglo-Indian Preventive Medicine, 1859-1914* (Cambridge: Cambridge University Press, 1994); Anil Kumar, *Medicine and the Raj: British Medical Policy in India, 1835-1911* (Walnut Creek, Calif.: Altamira, 1998); David Arnold, ed., *Imperial Medicine and Indigenous Societies* (Manchester: Manchester University Press, 1989); and Roy MacLeod and Milton Lewis, eds., *Diseases, Medicine, and Empire: Perspectives on Western Medicine and the Experience of European Expansion* (London: Routledge, 1988).

15. For exceptions to this tendency in British, French, and American historiography, see David Cantor, "Cortisone and the Politics of Empire: Imperialism and British Medicine," *Bulletin of the History of Medicine* 67 (1993): 463–93; Mark Harrison, "Tropical Medicine in Nineteenth-Century India," *British Journal of the History of Science* 25 (1992): 299–318; Maneesha Lal, "The Politics of Gender and Medicine in Colonial India: The Countess of Dufferin's Fund, 1885–1888," *Bulletin of the History of Medicine* 68 (1994): 29–66; Antoinette Burton, "Contesting the Zenana: The Mission to Make 'Lady Doctors for India,' 1874–1885," *Journal of British Studies* 35 (July 1996): 368–97; Michael Osborne, "Resurrecting Hippocrates: Hygienic Sciences and the French Scientific Expeditions to Egypt, Morea, and Algeria," in David Arnold (ed.), *Warm Climates and Western Medicine: The Emergence of Tropical Medicine, 1500-1900* (Amsterdam: Rodophi, 1996), 81–99; Patricia Lorcin, "Imperialism, Colonial Identity, and Race in Alge-

ria, 1830–1870: The Role of the French Medical Corps," *Isis* 90, no. 4 (December 2000): 653–79.

16. Antoinette Burton, "Rules of Thumb: British History and 'Imperial Culture' in Nineteenth- and Twentieth-Century Britain," *Women's History Review* 3, no. 4 (1994): 486.

17. The literature is growing, but representative works include John MacKenzie, *Propaganda and Empire* (Manchester: Manchester University Press, 1984); John MacKenzie, ed., *Imperial and Popular Culture* (Manchester: Manchester University Press, 1986); Annie E. Coombes, *Reinventing Africa: Museums, Imperial Culture, and Popular Imagination* (New Haven: Yale University Press, 1994); Edward Said, *Culture and Imperialism* (New York: Alfred A. Knopf, 1994); and Anne McClintock, *Imperial Leather: Race, Gender, and Sexuality in the Colonial Context* (London: Routledge, 1995).

18. See George Stocking, Jr., *Victorian Anthropology* (New York: Free Press, 1987); Henrika Kuklick, *The Savage Within: The Social History of British Anthropology, 1885–1945* (Cambridge: Cambridge University Press, 1991); Robert Stafford, *Scientist of Empire: Roderick Murchinson, Scientific Exploration, and Victorian Imperialism* (Cambridge: Cambridge University Press, 1989); Gauri Viswanathan, *Masks of Conquest: Literary Study and British Rule in India* (New York: Columbia University Press, 1989); Antoinette Burton, *Burdens of History: British Feminists, Indian Women, and Imperial Culture, 1865–1915* (Chapel Hill: University of North Carolina Press, 1994); Mrinalini Sinha, *Colonial Masculinity: The "Manly Englishman" and the "Effeminate Bengali" in the Late Nineteenth Century* (Manchester: Manchester University Press, 1995); Laura Tabili, *"We Ask for British Justice": Workers and Racial Difference in Late Imperial Britain* (Ithaca, N.Y.: Cornell University Press, 1994); Richard Grove, *Green Imperialism: Colonial Expansion, Tropical Island Edens, and the Origins of Environmentalism, 1600–1860* (Cambridge: Cambridge University Press, 1995); and Susan Thorne, *Congregational Missions and the Making of Imperial Culture in Nineteenth-Century England* (Stanford: Stanford University Press, 1999).

19. See paragraph 34, Medical Act of 1858 (21 & 22 Vict. c. 90).

20. See paragraph 36, Medical Act of 1858 (21 & 22 Vict. c. 90).

21. See Patrick Manson, "Introduction Address: On the Necessity for Special Education in Tropical Medicine," *Lancet*, 2 October 1897, 842; Terence J. Johnson and Marjorie Caygill, "The British Medical Association and Its Overseas Branches: A Short History," *Journal of Imperial and Commonwealth History* 1, no. 3 (May 1973): 304.

22. These rounded figures refer to the state and colonial services after midcentury: 900 in the Army Medical Department, 320 in the Colonial Medical Services, 700 in the Indian Medical Service, and 400 in the Naval Medical Service. On the army, see Sir Neil Cantlie, *A History of the Army Medical Department*, vol. 2 (Edinburgh: Churchill Livingstone, 1974), 269–70, 279, 284. On the Colonial Medical Service, see "Medical Appointments in the Colonies," *British Medical Journal*, 28 August 1897, 558–59; on the Indian Medical Service, see D. G. Crawford, *Roll of the Indian Medical Service, 1615–1930* (London: Thacker, 1930), appendix 9 [1865–1896], 639–41; and on the Naval Medical Department, see Christopher Lloyd and Jack L. S. Coulter, *Medicine and the Navy, 1815–1900*, vol. 4 (London: E. & S. Livingstone, 1963), 10.

23. E. B. van Heyningen, "Agents of Empire: The Medical Profession in the Cape

Colony, 1880–1910," *Medical History* 33 (1989): 450–71, and Diana Dyson, "The Medical Profession in Colonial Victoria, 1834–1901," in Roy MacLeod and Milton Lewis (eds.), *Disease, Medicine, and Empire; Perspectives on Western Medicine and the Experience of European Expansion* (London: Routledge, 1988), 194–209.

24. On this aspect of the profession, see Peterson, *Medical Profession in Mid-Victorian London*, 124–26; Digby, *Making a Medical Living*, 144–47; and Douglas M. Haynes, "Social Status and Imperial Status: Tropical Medicine and the British Medical Profession in the Nineteenth Century," in David Arnold (ed.), *Warm Climates and Western Medicine: The Emergence of Tropical Medicine, 1500–1900*, (Amsterdam: Rodophi, 1996), 208–20.

25. On overcrowding, see Haynes, "Social Status and Imperial Status," 215–20.

26. See chart 1 in Johnson and Caygill, "The British Medical Association and Its Overseas Branches," 308. Peter Bartrip largely overlooks the empire in his institutional history of the British Medical Association. See Bartrip, *Themselves Writ Large*, 292–300.

27. See Haynes, "Social Status and Imperial Status," 208–12.

28. For example, see "Medical Annotations: Physicians in China," *Lancet*, 7 April 1860, 355; "Eastern and European Medicine," *Lancet*, 24 November 1866, 582; "Native African Physic," *Lancet*, 29 December 1866, 732; and "Medicine as a Factor in Colonisation," *Lancet*, 27 April 1889, 852.

29. For a selection, see "[Editorial] How to Live in Tropical Climates," *Lancet*, 20 June 1863, 696–97; "The Health of the African Missions," *Lancet*, 1 August 1863, 137; "[Editorial] The Climate of the West Coast of Africa," *Lancet*, 28 November 1863, 626–27; "Europeans in Africa," *Lancet*, 15 October 1864, 442–43; "The Preservation of Life on the Congo," *Lancet*, 16 January 1886, 120; "[Editorial] Racial Pathology of Europeans in the Tropics," *Lancet*, 20 September 1890, 623–24; and Luigi Sambon, "Remarks on the Possibility of the Acclimatisation of Europeans in Tropical Regions," *British Medical Journal*, 9 January 1897, 61–65.

30. Burton, "Contesting the Zenana." See also Lal, "The Politics of Gender and Medicine in Colonial India."

Chapter 1. The Making of an Imperial Doctor

1. *Parish Church Marriage Register*, Church of Scotland, Old Machar.

2. Personal communication from A. Cameron, archivist of the Bank of Scotland.

3. Parish records, Oldmeldrum, Central Library, Aberdeen, Scotland.

4. Robert E. Tyson, "The Economy of Aberdeen," in John Smith and David Stevenson, eds., *Aberdeen in the Nineteenth Century: The Making of the Modern City* (Aberdeen: Aberdeen University Press, 1988), 20–22, 32.

5. St. Nicholas Parish, North: 1861 Census of Aberdeen.

6. University of Aberdeen, *Bursary Records*, nos. 206 (1860) and 105 (1861) for Forbes and no. 134 (1862) for David.

7. R. D. Anderson, *Education and Opportunity in Victorian Scotland: Schools and Universities* (Oxford: Clarendon Press, 1983), 5–6, 58–71. University of Aberdeen, "Abstract of the Medical Graduation Examination, November 2, 1861," in *Preliminary Education of Medical Students*, U.77, 16.

8. The Medical Act of 1858 (21 & 22 Vict. c. 90) contributed to the creation of a national medical profession, not only by placing Scottish and Irish examining and licensing bodies on the same footing with English institutions but also by extending the right of all duly qualified practitioners to practice medicine and surgery anywhere in the United Kingdom and the wider empire.

9. University of Aberdeen, *Graduate Schedules*, 1861–1870, U.61.

10. University of Aberdeen, *Second Professional Examination*, 20 July to August 1863, 42; *Third Professional Examination*, 25 July to 4 August 1864, 59, U.77.

11. Personal communication from Durham County archivist.

12. See entry for Patrick Manson in Col. William Johnston, "Aberdeen University: Roll of Graduates," *Aberdeen University Studies* 10 (1900): 640.

13. Manson-Bahr and Alcock, *Life and Work*, 3.

14. See Anne Digby, *Making a Medical Living: Doctors and Patients in the English Market for Medicine* (Cambridge: Cambridge University Press, 1994), 140–44, and M. Jeanne Peterson, *The Medical Profession in Mid-Victorian London* (Berkeley: University of California Press, 1978), 90–135.

15. See "Medical Appointments: Scotch Doctors and English Appointments," *Lancet*, 26 February 1859, 222, and "A New Kind of Scotch Doctor," *Lancet*, 21 April 1860, 406. See *British Parliamentary Papers*, "Report of the Select Committee on the Medical Act Amendment Bill and the Medical Appointments Qualifications Bill with Proceedings, and Minutes of Evidence," vol. 4 (1878–1880): 1370–74, 1471–77, 1485–88, 1590–93, 3051–52, 3330–34, 3358–68, 3863–70, 4026–35; *Brit. Parl. Papers*, "Report of the Select Committee of the House of Lords on Metropolitan Hospitals," vol. 16 (1890): 2504–15, 2641–44, 3596–3600, 9042–50, 9706–10; vol. 13 (1890–1891): 11, 177–79, 11,223–25, 15,351–57, 19,124–26.

16. This practice not only gave the metropolitan London-based Colleges a monopoly on appointments, but also enabled them to consolidate their power in the two key institutions of regular medicine: medical schools and hospitals. See Peterson, *Medical Profession in Mid-Victorian London*, 190–92.

17. Ibid., 85–86. Many Scottish practitioners simply complied. This is borne out by the geographical locations where fellows of the elite London corporations received their medical degrees. Between 1800 and 1889, 34 and 13 percent of the fellows of the Royal Colleges of Physicians and Surgeons, respectively, received their medical degrees from Scottish universities. See 51–52, Tables 1 and 2.

18. John Fairbank and Edwin O. Reischauer, *China: Tradition and Transformation* (New York: Houghton Mifflin, 1989), 277–89.

19. Manson-Bahr and Alcock, *Life and Work*, 5.

20. Lien-The Wu, *Plague Fighter: The Autobiography of a Modern Chinese Physician* (Cambridge, England: W. Heffer, 1959), 403–6.

21. The geographical mobility of Aberdeen graduates is based on locations reported in *Aberdeen Roll of Graduates* and the *Medical Directory for 1889 and 1899* (London: Churchill, 1890 and 1900). In addition, the mobility of Aberdeen graduates reflected wider behavior among non-English medical graduates in the United Kingdom. Scottish and Irish medical graduates dominated the medical professions in colonial Cape Town and Victoria. Between 1880 and 1909, Scottish degree holders outnumbered. English degree holders sixfold. For Victoria, the distribution of British qualifications among registered doctors between 1850 and 1901 included 654 Scottish, 92 Irish, 68 English, and

525 Australian university degrees. For Cape Colony, the distribution of licenses was as follows: 1,145 Scottish, 1,888 English, and 449 Irish. See Diana Dyason, "The Medical Profession in Colonial Victoria, 1834–1901," in M. Lewis and Roy MacLeod, eds., *Disease, Medicine, and Empire* (London: Routledge, 1989), 195–96, and E. B. van Heynigen, "The Medical Profession in Cape Colony," *Medical History* 33 (1989): 451.

22. William Mayers, N. B. Dennys, and Charles King, eds., *The Treaty Ports of China and Japan: A Complete Guide to the Open Ports of Those Countries, Together with Peking, Yedo, Hongkong, and Macao* (London: Trubner, 1867), appendix I, iii–iv.

23. J. D. Clark, *Formosa*, compiled from the *Shanghai Mercury* (Taipei: Ch'eung Wen, 1879), 91–95, 52–53.

24. For Manson's ship examinations, see *Formosa Diary*, 1865–1867, 8–24. This volume is held at the Library of the School of Hygiene and Tropical Medicine, University of London.

25. Clark, *Formosa*, 130–32.

26. Mayers, Dennys, and King, *Treaty Ports of China and Japan*, 247, 272–73.

27. Wu, *Plague Fighter*, 405.

28. See Robert L. Irick, *Ch'ing Policy toward the Coolie Trade, 1847-1878* Asian Library Series, no. 18. (San Francisco: Chinese Material Center, 1982).

29. Wu, *Plague Fighter*, 405.

30. "Medical Reports, No. 3," in *Imperial Chinese Customs Gazette* (Shanghai: Statistical Department of the Inspectorate General, 1872), 23; "Medical Reports, No. 4" (1873), 7; "Medical Reports, No. 5" (1873), 9.

31. Wu, *Plague Fighter*, 403, 406–7.

32. For Manson's role as physician to the consul general, Manson's application for medical adviser to Colonial Office to Sir Edward Wingfield, permanent undersecretary of state, Public Record Office CO 323/425/14027.

33. Daniel J. MacGowan, *Claims of the Missionary Enterprise on the Medical Profession* (New York: William Osborne, 1842), 13.

34. Rev. James Johnston, *China and Formosa: The Story of the Mission of the Presbyterian Church of England* (London: Hazell, Watson, and Viney, 1897), 93, 121, 387.

35. Theron Kue-Hing Young, "A Conflict of Professions: The Medical Missionary in China, 1835–1890," *Bulletin for the History of Medicine* 47 (1973): 259–60, 269–71.

36. MacGowan, *Claims of the Missionary Enterprise*, 23–24.

37. "Medical Annotations: Physicians in China," *Lancet*, 7 April 1860, 355.

38. "Eastern and European Medicine," *Lancet*, 24 November 1866, 582. On Western medical training, see also "Medical Education in China," *Lancet*, 31 July 1886, 222.

39. See Theron Kue-Hing Young, "A Conflict of Professions," 69.

40. *Report of the Amoy Missionary Hospital for 1871 (1872)*, 8,5. Sir Patrick Manson Archive, Personal and Biographical Papers, Life and Work, Contemporary Medical Archives, Wellcome Tropical Institute of Medicine, F.2, p. 5.

41. *Report of the Amoy Chinese Hospital for 1873* (1874), 2–3. Sir Patrick Manson Archive, Personal and Biographical Papers, F.4 Contemporary Medical Archives, Wellcome Tropical Institute. The title of the 1873 report reflected the hospital's name change of that year.

42. Ibid., 2, 3–4.

43. Ibid, 4.

44. Ibid, 6.

45. Paul Cohen, "Christian Missions and Their Impact to 1900," in John Fairbanks (ed.), *The Cambridge History of China*, vol. 10, *Late Ch'ing, 1800-1911*, pt. 1 (Cambridge: Cambridge University Press, 1978), 543–76.

46. Andrew Blake, "Foreign Devils and Moral Panics: Britain, Asia, and the Opium Trade," in Bill Schwartz, ed., *The Expansion of England: Race, Ethnicity and Cultural History* (New York: Routledge, 1996), 232–54.

47. Eli Chernin, "Sir Patrick Manson's Studies on the Transmission and Biology of Filariasis," *Reviews of Infectious Diseases* 5, no. 2 (March–April 1983): 359–60.

48. *RACH for the Year 1873* (1874), 4.

49. For this article, see Sir Patrick Manson, Personal and Biographical Papers, F.5. Contemporary Medical Archives, Wellcome Tropical Institute.

Chapter 2. Transforming Colonial Knowledge into Imperial Knowledge

1. See "Rules and Regulations," *The Colonial Office List for 1895* (London: Harrison, 1897), 334–35. Colonial medical officers in the West African colonies accrued six months of leave for every twelve months of service. See "Medical Appointments in the Colonies," *British Medical Journal*, 28 August 1897, 558. The interruption of leave was a regular grievance in the India Medical Service; see Mark Harrison, *Public Health in British India: Anglo-Indian Preventive Medicine, 1859-1914* (Cambridge: Cambridge University Press, 1994), 10–12.

2. Ann Stoler, "Making Empire Respectable: The Politics of Race and Sexual Morality in Twentieth-Century Colonial Cultures," in Jan Breman, ed., *Imperial Monkey Business: Racial Supremacy in Social Darwinist Theory and Colonial Practice* (Amsterdam: VU University Press, 1990), 35–64.

3. Hart described the expectations of imperial servants in the Service to his London agent, James Duncan Campbell: "Did you know that young v. Wurmb was about to marry? The first thing he said on arrival was to announce intention: I wired 'Postpone for three years,' but he decided otherwise. Tell all those who join in future that during their first period, seven years, they are not to marry." See Hart to Campbell, letter no. 1123, in John K. Fairbank, Katherine Frost Bruner, and Elizabeth MacLeod Matheson, eds., *The I.G. in Peking: Letters of Robert Hart, Chinese Maritime Customs, 1868-1907*, vol. 2 (Cambridge: Belknap Press of Harvard University, 1975), 1179.

4. Paul King, *In the Chinese Customs: A Personal Record of Forty-seven Years* (London: Fisher Unwin, 1924), 17–18.

5. William Fred Myers, N. B. Dennys, and Charles King, eds., *The Treaty Ports of China and Japan: A Complete Guide to the Open Ports of Those Countries, Together with Peking, Yedo, Hongkong and Macao* (London: Trubner, 1867), 261.

6. King, *In the Chinese Customs*, 18.

7. Ibid., 25. Early in his career, Hart described the opportunity for long-term relationships with Chinese women: "My salary wd not support an English wife: such a person is considered a great 'bother' out here: delicate—sickly—demanding great attention, medical care, and numerous servants, &c. &c.; such is the condition of an English lady

in China. Now some of the China women are very good looking: you can make one your absolute possession for from 50 to 100 dollars and support her at a cost of 2 or 3 dollars per month." See Hart's journal entry on 20 October 1854 in Katherine Frost Bruner, John K. Fairbank, and Richard J. Smith, eds., *Entering China's Service: Robert Hart's Journals, 1854-1863* (Cambridge: Harvard University Press, 1986), 71.

8. Hart's relationship with Ayaou began in late 1858 or early 1859 and produced three children. In 1866 he married Jane Bredon, who thereafter lived primarily in England while Hart continued his life in China. On Hart's romance with Ayaou, see Bruner et al., *Entering China's Service*, 151-54.

9. King, *In the Chinese Customs*, 25.

10. Even Manson could make exceptions. Paul King recalled, "Like most great doctors he did not always practise what he preached, and I remember on one occasion, after an eloquent exhortation against iced drinks on an empty stomach, seeing him empty almost at a draught a long glass, and they were long, of icy-beer just before sitting down to tiffin [lunch]. He beamed at us all and said, 'You young fellows mustn't do that.'" Ibid., 40.

11. "Medical Reports, No. 5," in *Imperial Chinese Customs Gazette* (Shanghai: Customs Press, 1873), 8.

12. Interview with Lady Manson, conducted by P. H. Manson-Bahr. Sir Patrick Manson Archive, F.7, box 11, Contemporary Medical Archives, Wellcome Institution for the History of Medicine.

13. "Medical Reports, No. 5," 7, 8.

14. Philippa Levine, "Venereal Disease, Prostitution, and the Politics of Empire: The Case of British India," *Journal of the History of Sexuality* 4, no. 4 (1994): 579-602. See also Antoinette Burton, *Burdens of History: British Feminists, Indian Women, and Imperial Culture, 1865-1915* (Chapel Hill: University of North Carolina Press, 1994), 127-69, and Kenneth Ballhatchet, *Race, Sex, and Class Under the Raj: Imperial Attitudes and Policies and Their Critics, 1793-1905* (London: Weidenfeld and Nicolson, 1980), 40-95.

15. Burton, *Burdens of History*, 130.

16. "Medical Reports, No. 5," 8.

17. On the role and function of white women in the empire, see Margaret Strobel, *European Women and the Second British Empire* (Bloomington: Indiana University Press, 1991).

18. See Philip H. Manson-Bahr and A. Alcock, *The Life and Work of Sir Patrick Manson* (London: Cassell, 1927), 38-39.

19. A. James Hammerton, *Emigrant Gentlewomen: Genteel Poverty and Female Emigration, 1830-1914* (London: Croom Helm, 1979), 28.

20. See Manson-Bahr and Alcock, *Life of Manson*, 38-39.

21. The description in this and the following four paragraphs is based on Ralph Muller and John R. Baker, *Medical Parasitology* (Philadelphia: J. B. Lippincott, 1990), 102-8.

22. "Medical Reports, No. 13," in *Imperial Chinese Customs Gazette* (Shanghai: Customs Press, 1872), 25-30.

23. For representative surgical examples, see James Irving, "Notes of a Case of Very Large Elephantiasis Scroti," *Indian Annals of Medical Science* 11 (1867): 405-7; James

Irving, "Case of Elephantiasis of the Scrotum," *Indian Annals of Medical Science* 19 (1865): 70–73; and Kenneth McLeod, "A Mirror of Hospital Practise: Case III — Scrotal Elephantiasis and Haematocele: Tapping: Inflammation and Soughing of Scrotum: Removal of Elephantoid Mass: Tetanus," *Indian Medical Gazette*, 1 December 1874, 325–26.

24. "Medical Reports, No. 13," 25, 26.

25. Ibid., 25, 26.

26. Ibid, 27–31. Anglo-Indian surgeons pioneered similar procedures and reported success. See Surgeon-Major H. Cayley, "Esmarch's 'Bloodless Method' Employed for the Excision of a Scrotal Tumour," *Indian Medical Gazette*, 1 May 1874, 131–32, and Surgeon-Major S. B. Patridge, "On the Bloodless Removal of Elephantoid Tumours of the Scrotum," *Indian Medical Gazette*, 1 January 1875, 13–14.

27. "Medical Reports, No. 5," 9–10, 14.

28. "The Week," *British Medical Journal*, 27 May 1865, 542.

29. See "Correspondence: The Indian Medical Gazette," *British Medical Journal*, 12 April 1884, 750. As late as 1898, conditions had not improved. Leonard Rodgers of the Indian Medical Service complained, "One of the greatest difficulties that those who work abroad have to contend with is that of access to the literature of tropical diseases. In fact it is not too much to say that a visit to England is in most cases necessary if the scattered references to any given disease have to be studied, and even prolonged search in one of the larger medical libraries of the metropolis will be entailed. It would, then, be of the greatest service to tropical medicine if a reference library could be started in connection with the *Journal of Tropical Medicine*." "The Need of a Library of Tropical Medicine," *Journal of Tropical Medicine*, December–January 1898, 144.

30. This point is made by Thomas Richards in *The Imperial Archive: Knowledge and the Fantasy of Empire* (London: Verso, 1993), 3–9, 13–17. For a general history of the British Museum, see Edward Miller, *That Noble Cabinet: A History of the British Museum* (London: Andre Deutsch, 1973).

31. At present, there is no comprehensive study on western medicine in the British empire.

32. Manson's reading notes during his furlough in 1874–1875 are included in his "Amoy Notebook." The notebook consists of 182 numbered pages and 2 without pagination. Page references refer to Manson's pagination. The "Amoy Notebook" is held by the Library of the School of Hygiene and Tropical Medicine, University of London.

33. Until recently, it was customary to view medicine in the empire as a backwater of medicine in Britain. But see Mark Harrison, "Tropical Medicine in Nineteenth Century India," *British Journal of the History of Science* 25 (1992): 299–318; Harrison, *Public Health in British India*; David Arnold, *Colonizing the Body: State Medicine and Epidemic Disease in Nineteenth-Century India* (Berkeley: University of California Press, 1993); and Anil Kumar, *Medicine and the Raj: British Medical Policy in India, 1835-1911* (Walnut Creek, Calif.: Altamira Press, 1998).

34. H. V. Carter, "On the Connection Between a Local Affection of the Lymphatic System and Chylous Urine with Remarks on the Pathology of the Disease," *Medico-Chirurgical Transactions* 45 (1862): 189–207, abstracted in "Amoy Notebook," 38–49. Manson also noted ("Amoy Notebook," 55) another publication on elephantiasis by Vandyke Carter, "On the Varix Lymphaticus: Its Coexistence with Elephantiasis: To Which Are Added, Remarks on the Pathology of the Last-Named Disease," *Transactions of the*

Medical and Physical Society of Bombay [Read December 1860 and December 1861], 171–200.

35. See Carter, "On the Connection Between a Local Affection of the Lymphatic System."

36. "Effects of Climate upon Man," *Colonial Magazine* 3 (1840): 165–73, 318–25; "Notices: Health of the Troops in India," *Madras Journal of Literature and Science* 15 (1848): 201; Francis Day, "On Tropical Diseases," *Lancet*, 16 January 1858, 58–60; [continued] 23 January 1858, 84–85; 13 March 1858, 261–62; and 3 April 1858, 337–38; James R. Martin, *The Influence of Tropical Climates on European Constitutions, Including Practical Observations on the Nature and Treatment of the Diseases of Europeans on Their Return from Tropical Climates* (London: J. Churchill, 1856); R. Clarke, "Remarks on the Topography and Diseases of the Gold Coast, West Africa," *Transactions of the Epidemiological Society* 1, no. 1 (1860): 76–128; William Smart, "Observations on the Climatology, Topography, and Diseases of Hong-Kong, and the Canton-River Station," Ibid. 1, no. 1 (1861): 191–228; James Horton, *The Diseases of Tropical Climates and Their Treatment* (London: J. Churchill, 1874, 1879).

37. Edward Waring, "On Elephantiasis, as It Exists in Travancore," *Indian Annals of Medical Science* 5 (January 1858): 1–15, quotation on p. 14. Abstracted in "Amoy Notebook," 83–90.

38. George Ballingall, "Surgical Cases and Observations," *Transactions of the Medical and Physical Society of Bombay* 4 (1858): 98–99. Abstracted in "Amoy Notebook," 98–99.

39. Charles Morehead, *Clinical Researches on Disease in India*, 2d ed. (London: Longman, Green, 1860), 699. Abstracted in "Amoy Notebook," 67.

40. Francis Day, "Elephantiasis Arabum, or 'Cochin Leg,'" *Madras Quarterly Journal of Medical Science* 1 (1860): 37–86, quotation on pp. 47–48. Abstracted in "Amoy Notebook," 109–11.

41. Vincent Richards, "Elephantiasis Arabum, Being a Sketch of the Disease as It Exists in Northern Orissa: Its Treatment and Influence on Opium-Eating," *Indian Annals of Medical Science* 9 (1873), reprinted in Tilbury Fox and T. Farquhar, eds., *On Certain Endemic Skin and Other Diseases of India and Hot Climates Generally* (London: J. Churchill, 1876), 126–47, quotation on p. 136. Abstracted in "Amoy Notebook," 115–22.

42. "Medical Reports, No. 13," Imperial *Chinese Customs Gazette*, part 6 (Shanghai: Customs Press, 1872), 24–25.

43. "Amoy Notebook," 109.

44. Kenneth McLeod, "Remarks on Varicose Lymphaticus or Naevoid Elephantiasis," *Indian Medical Gazette*, 1 August 1874, 204–08 and "Lewis on Nematode Haematozoa," *Indian Medical Gazette*, 1 February 1875, 46–47. For references to Lewis in Manson's notebook, see "Amoy Notebook", 122–23 and 125–7. On Lewis's career, see "Obituary: Timothy R. Lewis," *British Medical Journal*, 26 June 1886, 1242–43.

45. Timothy R. Lewis, *On a Haematozoa Inhabiting Human Blood: Its Relation to Chyluria and Other Diseases* (Calcutta: Office of the Superintendent of Government Printing, 1872), 6, 8, 40–41.

46. McLeod, "Remarks on Varicose Lymphaticus or Naevoid Elephantiasis," 207.

47. After two years, Lewis detected *filariae* in the blood of his original case. He reported that "... not only may those found in man *live for a period of more than 2½*

years, for certain, but that there is no evidence that they have any tendency to develop beyond a certain stage so long as they remain in circulation. For aught we know to the contrary, these Filariae may live for many years, and thus, at any moment, no matter how long after a previous attack, nor in what country the person may reside, he may be surprised by the sudden accession of Chyluria or any other obscure disease, such as will readily be understood by the physician when he becomes aware of the state of the blood." See Lewis, *On a Haematozoon Inhabiting the Human Blood*, 48.

48. Ibid., 27–28.

49. T. R. Lewis, "The Pathological Significance of Nematode Haematozoa," forming appendix B to the *Tenth Annual Report of the Sanitary Commissioner with the Government of India* (Calcutta, 1874), reprinted in Sir William Aitken, G. E. Dobson, and A. E. Brown, eds., *In Memoriam, Physiological and Pathological Researches; Being a Reprint of the Principal Scientific Writings of the Late T. R. Lewis* (London: Lewis Memorial Committee, 1888), 535, 539–45.

50. Johannes Japetus Steenstrup, *On the Alternative Generations; or the Propagation and Development of Animals through Alternate Generations: A Peculiar Form of Fostering Young in Lower Classes of Animals* (London: Ray Society, 1845). See also the informative articles by John Farley, "The Spontaneous Generation Controversy (1700–1860): The Origin of Parasitic Worms," *Journal of the History of Biology* 5, no. 1 (spring 1975): 95–125, and "Parasites and the Germ Theory of Disease," in Charles E. Rosenberg and Janet Golden, eds., *Framing Disease: Studies in Cultural History* (New Brunswick, N.J.: Rutgers University Press, 1992), 33–46.

51. Lewis, "The Pathological Significance of Nematode Haematozoa," 548.

52. Ibid., 546–47.

53. K. McLeod, "Lewis in Nematode Haematozoa," *Indian Medical Gazette*, 1 February 1874, 46.

54. Lewis deduced three likely sources of disease arising from the presence of *F. sanguinis hominis*. One was the pressure on vessels of tumors and nodules that enclosed worms. The perforation of tissue by the migration activity of the adult worm formed the second. A third source of interference was the congestion and subsequent rupturing of the delicate capillary walls, brought on by the activity of liberated ova. See Lewis, "Pathological Significance of Nematode Haematozoa," 555–56.

55. McLeod, "Lewis on Nematode Haematozoa," 47.

56. McLeod was not alone in his guarded endorsement. See Fox and Farquhar, *On Certain Endemic Skin and Other Diseases*, 36–41.

57. "Medical Reports, No. 10," *Imperial Chinese Customs Gazette*, part 6 (Shanghai: Customs Press, 1875), 1–12, quotation on page 6. This report was subsequently reprinted; see Patrick Manson, "Observations on Lymph-Scrotum and Allied Diseases," *Medical Times and Gazette*, 13 November 1875, 542–43, and 20 November 1875, 566–69.

58. Ibid, 10–11.

59. Ibid., 11.

60. Patrick Manson, "Observations on Lymph-Scrotum and Allied Diseases." Three years earlier, a notice on the medical reports of the Customs specifically referred to the report jointly authored by Manson and Muller ["Medical Reports, No. 13," 22–33]. See "Medicine in China," *Lancet*, 30 November 1872, 784.

61. On Manson's contact with T. B. Curling, see Thomas S. Cobbold, "Correspon-

dence: Discovery of the Intermediary Host of the *Filaria Sanguinis Hominis* (F. Bancrofti)," *Lancet*, 12 January 1878, 69. Curling discussed Manson's work on lymph scrotum and surgical technique for elephantiasis of the scrotum. See T. B. Curling, *A Practical Treatise on the Diseases of the Testis, and of the Spermatic Cord and Scrotum* (London: J. Churchill, 1878), 597, 613, 615–16. Excerpts from Manson's Customs report are referenced in Fox and Farquhar, *On Certain Endemic Skin and Other Diseases*, 36, 178–86, 196–202, 203–6.

62. See P. H. Manson-Bahr, *Patrick Manson: Father of Tropical Medicine* (London: Thomas Nelson, 1962), 4.

63. See William Aitken, *The Science and the Practise of Medicine* (London: Griffin, 1856 and 1860), 803.

64. "Medical Reports, No. 14," *Imperial Chinese Customs Gazette*, part 6 (Shanghai: Customs Press, 1877), 8.

65. "Medical Reports, No. 13," *Imperial Chinese Customs Gazette*, pt. 6 (Shanghai: Customs Press, 1877), 13–33. Lewis strongly recommended comparative study for prospective human *filaria* investigators: "Notwithstanding these minute anatomical discrepancies, which are of importance in considering the natural history of the two parasites, their resemblance is sufficiently striking, that I would strongly advise those who are interested in the human Haematozoon, and have not had the opportunity of examining it for themselves, but are anxious to obtain a more definite conception of the Filaria sanguinis hominis than can be obtained from written descriptions and drawings, to make arrangements with some of the low-caste persons employed in destroying sickly, pariah dogs, to collect a few ounces of blood of these animals." (See Lewis, "The Pathological Significance of Nematode Haematozoa," 539).

66. "Medical Reports, No. 13," 31.

67. "Medical Reports, No. 14" (Special Series No. 2), *Imperial Chinese Customs Gazette* (Shanghai: Customs Press, 1878), 1–6.

68. When describing the method of collecting specimens, Manson acknowledged that "to help in this work, which is excessively tedious and laborious, I familiarised two Chinese assistants with the appearance of the canine haematozoon, and showed them how to manipulate [the microscope] for the detection of similar organisms in man." "Medical Reports, No. 13," 31.

69. "Medical Reports, No. 14" (Special Series No. 2), *Imperial Chinese Customs Gazette* (Shanghai: Customs Press, 1878), 1–2, 5–6.

70. In alerting future investigators to the difficulty of searching for *filariae*, Manson offered his own experience: "I would warn others against a hasty examination of the blood, and against concluding that, because no filariae are found, none exist. For several years I have been in the habit of occasionally examining the discharge in lymph scrotum and the blood also, but until lately never encountered the *Filaria sanguinis hominis*. In fact, I kept a man for three or four years for the purpose of watching the progress of his lymph scrotum, and though I am convinced now that this man's blood contained filariae, yet, on account of my examining probably only a small part of one slide and with a high power, I always missed them" ("Medical Reports No. 13," 37).

71. Patrick Manson, *The Filaria Sanguinis Hominis and Certain Other New Forms of Parasitic Diseases in India, China, and Warm Countries* (London: H. K. Lewis, 1883), 10.

72. Hin-Lo is listed as number 46 in the clinical subject chart in Manson's epidemiological study of *filaria* in Amoy. See "Medical Reports, No. 14," 4, 9–10, 11.

73. Ibid, 10.

74. See Eli Chernin, "Sir Patrick Manson's Studies on the Transmission and Biology of Filariasis," *Reviews of Infectious Diseases* 5, no. 1 (January–February 1983): 148–63; John Farley, "Parasites and the Germ Theory of Disease," in Rosenberg and Golden, *Framing Disease*, 38–40; and François Delaporte, *The History of Yellow Fever: An Essay on the Birth of Tropical Medicine*, trans. Arthur Goldhammer (Cambridge: MIT Press, 1991), 20–25.

75. Muller and Baker, *Medical Parasitology*, 102–8.

76. He said as much in a later report: "Not all, but a very large proportion of the injected Filariae do thus *migrate*. My former observations were made entirely on Filariae found in the abdomen, or believed to be in the abdomen. Not suspecting this migration, and finding metamorphosis going on in the abdomen, I may have, unwittingly, included viscera of the former [that is, the thorax] in my examinations of the latter. On that occasion I traced out the metamorphosis to its conclusion, and entirely in what I thought, at the time, were abdominal tissues. It is likely, therefore, that migration to the thorax is not a necessary step indispensable for the welfare of the parasite. But, it is certainly the usual first step for the animal to take, and it is a fortunate one in the interests of the observer, as in tracing the subsequent steps of the metamorphosis, the ova, which in the abdomen are so annoying from their obscuring the field when ruptured, are not encountered. Lewis was the first to mention this migration; until I had read his description of his experiments on Filaria metamorphosis, I entirely overlooked this significant point." See Patrick Manson, "The Metamorphosis of *Filaria sanguinis hominis* in the Mosquito," *Journal of the Linnean Society of London (Zoology)*, 2d series, 2 (1884): 372.

77. In a footnote in a later report, Manson informed readers of the constructed nature of his "stages" of development: "The reader must bear in mind that this division of the metamorphosis is entirely artificial. No such thing exists in nature. What I describe as stages, in reality overlap each other; the gradations of development insensibly merge one into another." Ibid., 373.

78. "Medical Reports, No. 14," 11–12.

79. Ibid., 12.

80. Since the intermediary stage takes anywhere from ten days to three weeks—during which time the mosquito continues its feeding—it is almost certain that Manson starved his mosquitoes and the embryos to death. Joseph Bancroft, Jr., first suggested this defect in Manson's experimental practice. See Bancroft, "On the Metamorphosis of the Young Form of Filaria Bancrofti . . . in the Body of Culex Ciliaris, 'The House Mosquito of Australia,'" *Journal of Tropical Medicine*, 19 November 1899, 91–94.

81. Manson observed, "In one of these there was quite a number of embryos in regular gradation, from passive chrysalis up to the mature and very active embryo, so that there can be no doubt of the relationship of the latter to the former, though their appearances differ so much." See "Medical Reports, No. 14," 12–13.

82. Ibid., 13.

83. Ibid.

84. Ibid., 14.

Chapter 3. The Rhetoric and Politics of Discovery

1. See "The Week," *British Medical Journal*, 27 May 1865, 542; "Correspondence: The *Indian Medical Gazette*," *British Medical Journal*, 12 April 1884, 750; and Leonard Rodgers, "The Need of a Library of Tropical Medicine," *Journal of Tropical Medicine*, December–January 1898, 144.

2. P. W. J. Bartrip overlooks the empire in his institutional history of the *British Medical Journal*. See P. W. J. Bartrip, *Mirror of Medicine: The British Medical Journal* (Oxford: Clarendon Press for the British Medical Association, 1990).

3. "Obituary: T. Spencer Cobbold," *Lancet*, 27 March 1886, 616–17. He also held the Swiney Lectureship on Geology at the British Museum, which was opened only to graduates of medicine of the University of Edinburgh.

4. Thomas S. Cobbold, "Parasites and Their Strange Uses," lecture delivered in the Memorial Hall, Manchester, 12 November 1873, 45. See also Graeme Gooday, " 'Nature' in the Laboratory: Domestication and Discipline with the Microscope in Victorian Life Science," *British Journal of the History of Science*, 24 (1991): 307–41.

5. Thomas S. Cobbold, *Worms: A Series of Lectures on Practical Helminthology* (Philadelphia: Lindsay and Blakiston, 1872), 10.

6. For the most extensive discussion of the history of this disease, see John Harley, *Bilharzia: A History of Imperial Tropical Medicine* (Cambridge: Cambridge University Press, 1991), 48–50.

7. Ibid, 5, 54–56.

8. Thomas S. Cobbold, "On the Development of Bilharzia Haematobia," *British Medical Journal*, 27 June 1872 89.

9. Ibid., 89–92.

10. Ibid, 92.

11. Ibid. On Salisbury, See also Douglas D. Cunningham, "The Haematozoon: Notes on Its Discovery and Relation to *Canine Filaria*," *Lancet*, 14 June 1873, 835–36.

12. Cobbold, "On the Development of Bilharzia Haematobia," 92.

13. Mark Harrison, *Public Health in British India: Anglo-Indian Preventive Medicine, 1859-1914* (Cambridge: Cambridge University Press, 1994), 105–9.

14. "Obituary: Timothy Richards Lewis," *British Medical Journal*, 20 June 1886, 1242.

15. "The Fungoid Theory of Cholera," *British Medical Journal*, 12 November 1870, 535–36.

16. "Sanitary Work in India, No. II," *Lancet*, 17 December 1870, 858.

17. "Chylous Urine," *British Medical Journal*, 19 November 1870, 559.

18. "Worms in Urine and Blood," *Lancet*, 31 August 1872, 310.

19. "The Newly Discovered Haematozoon," *Lancet*, 21 December 1872, 889–90 and "The Haematozoon," *Lancet*, 11 January 1873, 56–57.

20. "Haematozoa and Chyluria," *British Medical Journal*, 8 February 1873, 147.

21. Ibid., 147–48. For a similar assessment of Lewis's comparative research on canine *filariae*, see "The Pathological Significance of Nematode Haematozoa," *Lancet*, 6 February 1875, 209–10, and "The Pathological Significance of Nematode Haematozoa," *Medical Times and Gazette*, 13 February 1875, 173–74.

22. Douglas M. Haynes, "Social Status and Imperial Service: Tropical Medicine and

the British Medical Profession in the Nineteenth Century," in David Arnold, ed., *Warm Climates and Western Medicine: The Emergence of Tropical Medicine, 1500-1900* (Amsterdam: Rodolpi, 1996), 211–15. On the Indian Medical Service, see Harrison, *Public Health in British India*, 6–35.

23. "Obituary: Timothy R. Lewis," 1242–43; Timothy R. Lewis, *On a Haematozoon Inhabiting Human Blood: Its Relation to Chyluria and Other Diseases* (Calcutta: Office of the Superintendent of Government Printing, 1872), 5. See also "Haematozoa and Chyluria," *British Medical Journal*, 8 February 1873, 147.

24. D. D. Cunningham, "The Haematozoon: Notes on Its Discovery and Its Relation to the Canine Filaria," *Lancet*, 14 June 1873, 835–37; Francis Welch, "On A Species of Filaria Found in the Interior of the Vascular System of a Dog: Relative to the Filaria in the Blood, and the Ova and Larvae of a Nematoid Worm in the Urine, of Man," *Lancet*, 8 March 1873, 336–38. Welch refers to Lewis's report in the appendix to the *Annual Report of the Sanitary Commissioners of India, 1871*.

25. Cunningham, "The Haematozoon," 835–36.

26. Ibid, 836.

27. Francis H. Welch, "The Haematozoon," *Lancet*, 28 June 1873, 905–6.

28. T. R. Lewis, "The Pathological Significance of Nematode Haematozoa," *Lancet*, 6 February 1875, 209–10.

29. Thomas S. Cobbold, "Fresh Discoveries by Dr. Lewis," *Lancet*, 6 February 1875, 216–17.

30. Thomas S. Cobbold, "Verification of Recent Haematozoal Discoveries in Australia and Egypt," *British Medical Journal*, 24 June 1876, 780–81. Cobbold made the same assertion about the nematoids in other articles: see "On Filaria Bancrofti," *Lancet*, 6 October 1877, 495–96; "Filaria Sanguinis Hominis," *Lancet*, 13 July 1878, 64; and "Medical Society of London: Filaria Sanguinis Hominis," *Lancet*, 30 March 1878, 465. Cobbold did not entirely misrepresent Sonsino's view: "However, Dr. Sonsino is convinced that the filariae found by him are not of the same species as the filaria sanguinis hominis of Lewis" ("Verification," 780).

31. Thomas S. Cobbold, "Discovery of the Adult Representative of Microscopic Filariae," *Lancet*, 14 July 1877, 70–71.

32. As cited in ibid., 70.

33. Ibid., 71.

34. Timothy R. Lewis, "*Filaria Sanguinis Hominis* (Mature Form) Found in a Blood-Clot in *Naevoid Elephantiasis* of the Scrotum," *Lancet*, 20 September 1877, 453–55. To prevent any suggestion that Prospero's find in Egypt was identical to his, Lewis added, "No sac has been observed surrounding such embryos in the blood of dogs, nor in those found in man in Egypt."

35. Ibid, 455.

36. "Obituary: T. Spencer Cobbold," *Lancet*, 27 March 1886, 616–17.

37. Thomas S. Cobbold, "On *Filaria Bancrofti*," *Lancet*, October 6, 1877, 495–96.

38. Ibid. Lewis drew attention to this rhetorical sleight of hand in one of Cobbold's many research reviews. See Thomas S. Cobbold, "Correspondence: Filaria Sanguinis Hominis," *Lancet*, 13 July 1878, 64. Cobbold described Bancroft as the discoverer of the adult representative even though Lewis had provided the most complete description earlier. "It is possible that the description supplied by Dr. Bancroft, which is quoted on a

previous page, is not considered sufficiently precise to be accepted as such, from a naturalist's point of view. Allowing this, if, as Dr. Cobbold maintains, the Australian and Indian parasites are identical, the first full account of the mature Filaria sanguinis hominis, as found in India, was published, both in this country and in London, previous to the appearance of Dr. Cobbold's description—having, indeed, been in the printer's hands before Dr. Cobbold had even seen the Australian parasites. Dr. Cobbold, moreover, refers to such prior publication in the appendix to his own article. . . . This trifling oversight will, I have no doubt, be duly corrected should this distinguished observer have occasion to write regarding these subjects in the future." Timothy R. Lewis, "The Nematoid Haematozoa of Man," *Quarterly Journal of Microscopical Science*, new series, 74 (April 1879): 258.

39. Thomas S. Cobbold, "Prof. T. S. Cobbold on the Life-History of *Filaria Bancrofti*," *Proceedings of the Linnean Society (Zoology)*, n.s. 14 (1878): 364.

40. Thomas S. Cobbold, "Discovery of the Intermediary Host of *Filaria Sanguinis Hominis (F. Bancrofti)*," *Lancet*, 12 January 1878, 69.

41. Ibid. Cobbold announced the discovery of the intermediary host at a meeting of the Pathological Society. See "Reports of Societies: The Pathological Society," *Medical Times and Gazette*, 16 March 1878, 291.

42. Manson-Bahr and Alcock, *Life and Work of Patrick Manson*, 56.

43. Lewis, "The Nematoid Haematozoa of Man."

44. See reference to initial report in "Is the Mosquito the Intermediary Host of the *Filaria Sanguinis Hominis?*" *British Medical Journal*, 22 June 1878, 904.

45. Lewis, "The Nematoid Haematozoa of Man," 251–52.

46. Ibid, 252.

47. Ibid, 252–253.

48. *British Medical Journal*, 22 June 1878, 904. This was an abstract of Lewis's report in the *Proceedings of the Asiatic Society of Bengal*. Lewis published a more comprehensive review of the literature, including Manson's discovery; see "The Nematoid Haematozoa of Man."

49. "The Development of the *Filaria Sanguinis Hominis*," *Medical Times and Gazette*, 7 September 1878, 275.

50. "Book Review: Organisms Found in the Blood of Man and Animals, and Their Relation to Disease," *Nature*, 15 May 1879, 76–77.

51. Cobbold, "*Filaria Sanguinis Hominis*," *Lancet*, 13 July 1878, 64.

52. Thomas S. Cobbold, "Prof. T. S. Cobbold on the Life-History of the Filaria Bancrofti," *Proceedings of the Linnean Society of London (Zoology)*, new series (1878): 356–68. Vol. 14

53. Patrick Manson, "Medical Reports, No. 14" (Special Series No. 2), *Imperial Chinese Maritime Customs* (Shanghai: Statistical Department of the Inspectorate General, 1878), 13. Cobbold also communicated this paper to the Linnean Society. See "Dr. Manson on the Development of *Filaria Sanguinis Hominis*," *Proceedings of the Linnean Society of London*, n.s., 14 (1878): 310.

54. Patrick Manson, "The Metamorphosis of the Filaria Sanguinis Hominis in the Mosquito" [communicated by Thomas S. Cobbold], *Journal of the Linnean Society (Zoology)* 2 (1884): 376.

55. Patrick Manson, "Original Communications: The Development of the *Filaria Sanguinis Hominis*," *Medical Times and Gazette*, 28 December 1878, 731.

56. Manson, "Medical Reports, No. 14," 1–2, 7.

57. Patrick Manson, "Medical Reports, No. 18" (Special Series No. 2), *Imperial Chinese Customs Gazette* (Shanghai: Statistical Department of the Inspectorate General, 1880), 36.

58. Ibid., 37, 39.

59. Thomas S. Cobbold, "Observations on *Filariae* by Drs. Patrick Manson, John R. Somerville, Joseph Bancroft, J. F. Da Silva Lima, J. L. Paterson, Pedro S. De Magalhaes, and J. Mortimer-Granville, communicated, with an Introduction, by the President," *Journal of the Queckett Microscopical Society*, 6 (1879–81): 66–71; "Further Observations on *Micro-Filariae*, with Description of New Species, (with a Prefatory Note] by the President)" [read June 25, 1880], *Journal of the Queckett Microscopial Society*, 130–40; "On the Periodicity of Filarial Migrations to and from the Circulation" (communicated by Dr. Cobbold) [read January 28, 1881], *Journal of the Queckett Microscopial Society*, 239–48.

60. Thomas S. Cobbold, "Observations on *Filariae*, . . . communicated, with an Introduction, by the President" [read February 27, 1880], *Journal of the Queckett Microscopial Society*, 59.

61. Ibid, 61.

62. "*Filariae* and the Febrile State," *Lancet*, 20 August 1881, 350–51; "Further Observations on *Micro-Filariae*"; "On the Periodicity of Filarial Migrations"; and Stephen Mackenzie, "X. Miscellaneous Specimens: A Case of Filarial Haemato-chyluria," *Transactions of the Pathological Society of London*, 33 (1882): 394–402.

63. See entry for Stephen Mackenzie in *The Concise Dictionary of National Biography* (Oxford: Oxford University Press, 1992), 2: 1893. Mackenzie was not alone. Tilbury Fox and T. Farquhar, the two leading metropolitan skin specialists, edited a book on skin diseases in India. See *On Certain Endemic Skin and Other Diseases of India and Hot Climates Generally* (London: J. Churchill, 1876).

64. Patrick Manson [communicated by George Thin], "Miscellaneous Specimens: Filaria in Lymph-Scrotum," *Transactions of the Pathological Society* 33 (1882): 285–302. Thin began his career in Shanghai after graduating from Edinburgh. He returned to Britain to become a respected dermatologist, specializing in tropical diseases. During the course of his career he published widely and advised shipping companies and other businesses in the Far East. See entry for George Thin in Bill Bynum and Caroline Overy (eds.), *The Beast in the Mosquito: The Correspondence of Ronald Ross and Patrick Manson* (Amsterdam: Rodophi, 1998), 505.

65. Patrick Manson, "Miscellaneous Specimens," 289–91.

66. Stephen Mackenzie, "X. Miscellaneous Specimens: 1. A Case of Filarial Haemato-Chyluria," *Transactions of the Pathological Society of London* 33 (1882): 394–410.

67. Ibid.

68. "Medical Societies: Pathological Society of London," *Lancet*, 22 October 1881, 707–9; "Annotations: *Filaria Sanguinis Hominis*," *Lancet*, 22 October 1881, 722–23.

69. Mackenzie, "Miscellaneous Specimens," 402.

70. "Pathological Society of London," 708.

71. "Annotations: *Filaria Sanguinis Hominis*," 722.

72. For references to the exhibit, see "Pathological Society of London," 708. Mac-

kenzie acknowledged Cobbold's assistance directly: "By the kindness of Dr. Cobbold I was able to exhibit to the Society mosquitoes containing embryo filariae from India, China, and Australia, and thus to demonstrate the role of the mosquito, and the identity of the filariae from widely different parts of the globe." See "A Case of Filarial Haematochyluria," 402.

73. "Pathological Society of London," 708.

74. "Annotations: *Filaria Sanguinis Hominis*," 722.

75. Shortly after the validation of Manson's discovery, two reports on biting experiments in Formosa (Taiwan), by Dr. Myers of the Customs Service and Prospero Sonsino of Egypt, were published. If anything, these experiments refined Manson's discovery by stressing that only certain species of mosquitoes hosted the *filaria* worm. "*Filaria Sanguinis Hominis*," *Lancet*, 10 December 1881, 1015–16; Prospero Sonsino, "A New Series of Cases of *Filaria Sanguinis* Parasitism Observed in Egypt," *Medical Times and Gazette*, 22 September 1883, pt. 1, 340–42, 29 September 1883, pt. 1 (cont.), 367–69, and 21 October 1883, pt. 2, 421–23.

76. Patrick Manson, "The Metamorphosis of *Filaria sanguinis hominis in the Mosquito*" [communicated by Thomas S. Cobbold], *Journal of the Linnean Society of London (Zoology)*, n.s., 2 (1884): 367–68.

77. Ibid., 368.

78. Ibid, 369.

79. Ibid, 373.

80. Ibid., 379.

81. "Notes and Memoranda: The Life-History of *Filaria Bancrofti*," *Journal of the Royal Microscopical Society* 1 (1878): 377; "Prof. T. S. Cobbold on the Life-History of *Filaria Bancrofti*," *Proceedings of the Linnean Society of London [Zoology)*, n.s., 14 (1878): 366; "Observations on Filariae," *Journal of the Queckett Microscopical Society* 6 (1879–81): 61; "Correspondence: Filaria Sanguinis Hominis," *Lancet*, 13 July 1878, 64; and Cobbold, *Parasites: A Treatise* (London: J. Churchill, 1879), 192–93.

82. Bourel-Roncière, "Pathologie Exotica: De L'Haematozoaire," *Archive de Médicine Navale* 30 (1878): 192–214.

83. Maurice Nielly, *Elements de Pathologie Exotique* (Paris: Adrien De la Hage et Emile Lecrosnier, 1881), 360–72.

84. "The Dipterous Enemies of Man," in Robert H. Lamborn (ed.), *Dragon Flies vs. Mosquitoes: Can the Mosquito Pest Be Mitigated?* (New York: D. Appleton, 1890), 52–53.

85. Alphonse Laveran, *De paludisme et de son haematozoaire* (Paris: Masson, 1891), 86–87.

86. "Book Review: *Filaria Sanguinis Hominis* and Certain New Forms of Parasitic Diseases," *British Medical Journal*, 26 April 1884, 821.

87. "Book Review: *Filaria Sanguinis Hominis* and Certain New Forms of Parasitic Diseases," *Veterinarian*, March 1883, 1.

88. Interview with Lady Manson, conducted by P. H. Manson-Bahr. Manson Archive, F7, box 11, Contemporary Medical Archives, Wellcome Institute for the History of Medicine.

89. He was estimated to have expected a comfortable £3,000–4,000 per year when he retired to Kildrummie, Scotland. See biographical materials, Manson Archive, F7, box 11, Contemporary Medical Archives, Wellcome Institute for the History of Medicine.

90. Manson-Bahr and Alcock, *Life and Work of Patrick Manson*, 81–85.

91. Patrick Manson, "Presidential Address," *Transactions of the Hong Kong Medical Society* (1889), 23–25.

92. In 1894, Manson was admitted to the fellowship of the College. See Manson-Bahr and Alcock, *Life and Work of Sir Patrick Manson*, 86, 125–26.

Chapter 4. Making Imperial Science British Science

1. See "Medical Annotations: The Encouragement of Scientific Research," *Lancet*, 28 November 1863, 627; Charles Babbage, *Reflections on the Decline of Science in England and on Some of Its Causes* (London: B. Fellowes, 1830); and Babbage, "The Exposition of 1851; or, Views of the Industry, the Science, and the Government of England" (1851), in Martin Campbell-Kelly (ed.), *The Works of Charles Babbage*, 11 vols. (London: William Pickering, 1989), 10:90–120. On the politics of public support for science funding, see Roy M. Macleod, "Resources of Science in Victorian England: The Endowment of Science Movement, 1868–1900," in Peter Mathias (ed.), *Science and Society, 1600–1900* (Cambridge: Cambridge University Press, 1972), 111–31. For an institutional account, see Peter Alter, *The Reluctant Patron: Science and the State in Britain, 1850–1920*, trans. Angela Davies (Oxford: New York, 1987).

2. Patrick Manson, "On the Nature and Significance of the Crescentic and Flagellated Bodies in Malarial Blood," *British Medical Journal*, 8 December 1894, 1306–8.

3. "Section of Tropical Diseases: The Mosquito and the Malarial Parasite," *British Medical Journal*, 24 September 1898, 849–53.

4. The description of the biology of the *Plasmodium falciparum* parasite is based on Milton J. Friedman and William Trager, "The Biochemistry of Resistance to Malaria," in Thomas D. Brock (ed.), *Readings from* Scientific American: *Microorganisms, from Smallpox to Lyme Disease* (New York: W. H. Freeman, 1990), 93–106.

5. Julius Mannaberg, *The Malaria Parasite: A Description Based upon Observations Made by the Author and Other Observers*, trans. R. W. Felkin (London: New Sydenham Society of London, 1894), 245–46.

6. Alphonse Laveran, *Traité des Fièvres Palustres* (Paris: Masson, 1884), 455–56. The failure to confirm the role of the parasite using Pasteur's bacteriological method placed Laveran on the defensive. "The beautiful work of M. Pasteur on anthrax and on cholera of chickens, has made the method of cultivation an honour, and it seems today, to read some authors, that all sickness ought to be submitted to this mode of experimentation" (452). In reference to his discovery, Laveran added, "We are in the presence of microbes of a very special morphology, which we are unable to confuse with common species; these microbes are absolutely specific to malaria, and their presence in the blood capillaries are tied more constantly to the pathological alterations of malaria" (452).

7. Dale C. Smith and Lorraine B. Sanford, "Laveran's Germ: The Reception and Use of a Medical Discovery," *Journal of Tropical Medicine and Hygiene*, 34(1) (1985): 2–20.

8. But the "bacillus" was quickly discredited. In fact, Sternberg was the first to publicly cast doubt on its role. See George Sternberg, "The Malarial 'Germ' of Laveran," *Medical Record*, 1 May 1886, 486. The news traveled quickly. See "The Malarial Poison,"

British Medical Journal, 19 November 1881, 827; "Bacillus Malariae," *British Medical Journal*, 10 December 1881, 935; Sir Joseph Fayrer, "Croonian Lectures on the Climate and Fevers of India," Lecture no. 2, *British Medical Journal*, 25 March 1882, 413–15; "Correspondence: The Bacillus Malariae," *British Medical Journal*, 19 August 1882, 342; and "The Organisms of Malaria," *Lancet*, 17 June 1882, 993–94.

9. Smith and Sanford, "Laveran's Germ," 10.

10. Laveran, *Traité des Fièvres Palustres*, 452, 456.

11. Ibid, 456.

12. Mannaberg, *The Malaria Parasite*, 413.

13. As early as 1881, George Sternberg discredited the role of the *Bacillus malariae* in causing malaria disease. See "Sternberg on the Etiology of Malarial Fevers," *London Medical Record*, 15 December 1881, 488–89.

14. Ettore Marchiafava and Angelo Celli, "Further Researches on Malaria," *Lancet*, 2 January 1886, 29.

15. Mannaberg, *The Malaria Parasite*, 247–49.

16. Ibid., 248–49.

17. Smith and Sanford, "Laveran's Germ," 12–13; George Sternberg, "The Malarial 'Germ' of Laveran, Parts I and II," *Medical Record*, 1 May 1886 and 8 May 1886, 489–93, 517–18. After some initial doubt, William Osler of Johns Hopkins University took up the cause of the *plasmodium* as well. See "News of the Week: 'Bacillus of Malaria Found at Last,'" *Medical Record*, 4 September 1886, 633–34, and "The Bacillus of Malaria," *British Medical Journal*, 15 January 1887, 121.

18. "British Medical Association: Micro-organisms Associated with Malaria," *Lancet*, 20 August 1887, 373.

19. "Parasites in Malaria," *Lancet*, 1 August 1891, 246.

20. "The International Congress of Hygiene and Demography," *Nature*, 15 January 1891, 241–42.

21. "The International Congress of Hygiene and Demography," *Times* (London), 8 August 1891, 8.

22. At the opening of the Congress, *Nature* stated, "Never before, perhaps, in the history of science has there been assembled together such a numerous gathering of eminent men of science of different nationalities, or representing so many countries, for the purpose of discussing scientific problems." See "The International Congress of Hygiene and Demography," *Nature*, 13 August 1891, 344.

23. "International Congress of Hygiene and Demography: Section II: Bacteriology," *British Medical Journal*, 15 August 1891, 358–59.

24. Charles-Louis-Alphonse Laveran, "De L'Haematozoa du Paludisme," in *Transactions of the Seventh International Congress of Hygiene and Demography*, 13 vols. (London: Erye and Spottiswoode, 1892), 7: 14–15, 17, 18.

25. W. North, "Haematozoa of Malaria," *Lancet*, 15 August 1891, 376.

26. Laveran, "De l'Haematozoa du Paludisme," 19, 20, 18.

27. For reports on the Congress, see *British Medical Journal*, 15 August 1891, 359, and *Lancet*, 15 August 1891, 375–76. For Manson's paper, see "The Geographical Distribution, Pathological Relation, and Life-History of *Filaria sanguinis diurna* and *Filaria sanguinis hominis* in Connection with Preventive Medicine," *British Medical Journal*, 15 August 1891, 373.

28. See Laveran's English abstract, "The Haematozooon of Malaria," in *Abstracts of Papers Communicated to the Seventh International Congress on Hygiene and Demography* (Eyre and Spottiswoode, 1891), 37–38.

29. Patrick Manson, "Malaria, and Its Associated Parasite," *Transactions of the Hunterian Society* (1894–95): 43–44.

30. On Manson's appointment, see *Minute Book of the Seamen's Hospital Society*, 25 March 1892, 125–26, and 10 June 1892, 141–44.

31. It was for this reason that Laveran advised would-be investigators "to repeat the examination of the blood several times before declaring the examination to be negative." See Alphonse Laveran, *Du paludisme and de son haematozoaire* (Paris: Masson, 1891), 35–36.

32. From a paper given before the Epidemiological Society of London on African Haemoglobinuric Fever in March 1893, it is clear that Manson was familiar with Laveran's parasite but had not detected it. "It would be easy to say, that malaria is the plasmodium malariae, or Laveran's bodies, and that malarial disease is an outcome of the action of these on the human body. This may be a perfectly correct definition, and in time it may prove to be such; but as yet it is premature." See "On African Haemoglobinuric Fever," *Transactions of the Epidemiological Society of London*, n.s., 12, session (1892–93): 113. On Manson's report of detection in the fall of 1893, see "Malaria, and Its Associated Parasite," 44.

33. Manson, "Malaria," 19–41; "A Clinical Lecture on the Parasite of Malaria and Its Demonstration," *British Medical Journal*, 6 January 1894, 6–9, and "Other Metropolitan Medical Societies: North London Medical and Chirurgical Society," *Lancet*, 24 March 1894: 744.

34. "Dr. Patrick Manson's Malaria Chart," *British Medical Journal*, 1 December 1894, 1252–54. Besides being a visible expert of the *plasmodium*, Manson was also the most vigorous defender of the existence of the plasmodia. On Manson's running dispute with Suregon-Colonel Lawrie of the Indian Medical Service, who doubted the existence of the malaria parasite, see "Condition of the Blood in Malaria," London *Times*, 6 August 1895, 3; "Correspondence: Malarial Parasite in the Blood," *British Medical Journal*, 10 August 1895, 394; "Correspondence: The Malarial Parasite," *British Medical Journal*, 24 August 1895: 503–4; and "Correspondence: The Malarial Parasite," *British Medical Journal*, 31 August 1895: 560.

35. See note on Ronald Ross's handwritten copy of his Parkes Prize essay. Item RA05/19, Ronald Ross Archive, London School of Hygiene and Tropical Medicine, University of London.

36. Manson, "Malaria, and Its Associated Parasite," 21.

37. Mannaberg, *The Malaria Parasite*, 289.

38. Ibid., 271–72.

39. Patrick Manson, "A Clinical Lecture on the Parasite of Malaria and Its Demonstration," 8–9.

40. Patrick Manson, "On the Nature and Significance of the Crescentic and Flagellated Bodies in Malarial Blood," *British Medical Journal*, 8 December 1894, 1307.

41. Alphonse Charles Laveran, *Paludism*, translated from French by J. W. Martin (London: New Sydenham Society, 1893).

42. Julius Mannaberg, *The Malaria Parasite: A Description Based upon Obser-

vations Made by the Author and Other Observers, translated from German by R. W. Felkin (London: New Sydenham Society of London, 1894).

43. Review, *British Medical Journal*, 27 October 1894, 924.

44. Laveran, *Traité des Fièvres*, 457.

45. Laveran, *Paludism*, 97–98, 96. For Bourel-Roncière, see "Pathologie Exotique: De L'Hematozoaire," *Archive de Médicine Navale*, 30 (1878):192–214.

46. See Mannaberg, *The Malaria Parasite*, 271.

47. Ibid., 284.

48. Ibid., 413.

49. Mannaberg was Manson's source of information regarding the failed mosquito infection experiments conducted by Grassi and Calandruccio. Ibid., 413.

50. Patrick Manson, "The Goulstonian Lectures on the Life-History of the Malaria Germ Outside the Human Body, No. III," *British Medical Journal*, 28 March 1896, 714.

51. Manson, "On the Nature and Significance of the Crescentic and Flagellated Bodies in Malarial Blood," 1306–7.

52. Ibid., 1306, 1307.

53. Ibid., 1307.

54. Ibid., 1308.

55. Ibid.

56. Ronald Ross, *Memoirs, with a Full Account of the Great Malaria Problem and Its Solution* (London: John Murray, 1923), 162–63.

57. Ibid., 126. See Ronald Ross, "The True Nature of the Plasmodium and the Malaria Parasite," *Indian Medical Gazette*, October 1893, 329–36, and "The third element of the blood and the malaria parasite," *Indian Medical Gazette*, January 1894, 5–14.

58. Ross, *Memoirs*, 109.

59. Ronald Ross, *Memories of Patrick Manson* (London: Harrison and Sons, 1930), 11–12.

60. Ross, *Memoirs*, 126–27.

61. Letter no. 1, Manson to Ross, 9 April 1894, in W. E. Bynum and Caroline Overy (eds.), *The Beast in the Mosquito: The Correspondence of Ronald Ross and Patrick Manson* (Amsterdam: Rodopi, 1998), 1. Unless otherwise noted, all references to the Ross and Manson correspondence will be from this volume.

62. Ross, *Memoirs*, 127.

63. Ibid., 127–29.

64. Ronald Ross, Parkes Prize essay, 12–13. Ronald Ross Archives, London School of Hygiene and Tropical Medicine.

65. Ross, *Memoirs*, 199–200. According to Ross, he spent the first three years as a regimental officer on unemployed pay. Letter No. 178 02/117, Ross to Manson, 20 June 1897, 200.

66. Ross, *Memoirs*, 134.

67. Letter no. 3 02/065, Ross to Manson, 15 May 1895, 7.

68. Letter no. 11 02/004, Manson to Ross, 21 June 1895, 31–32.

69. Letter no. 4 02/066, Ross to Manson, 22 May 1895, 11.

70. Ibid., 12.

71. Letter no. 13 02/005, Manson to Ross, 28 June 1895, 36–38.

72. Ross, *Memoirs*, 164. "I am nearly wild," Ross wrote on 17 July 1895, "and have

been able to do nothing for nearly six weeks now. I have been all round the hospitals again and have touts out everywhere and, with great difficulty have obtained three bazaar people—no crescents. The bazaar people won't come to me even though I offer what is enormous payment to them. I offer them 2 and 3 rupees for a single finger prick and much more if I find crescents—they think it is witchcraft." Letter no. 14, 02/072, Ross to Manson, 17 July 1895, 39.

73. "The Malaria Parasite," *Lancet*, 3 August 1895, 302.

74. Ibid. On Thin's familiarity with Manson's *filaria* research, see Patrick Manson, "Lymph Scrotum, Showing Filaria in Situ" [communicated by G. Thin], *Transactions of the Pathological Society* (1881): 285–302.

75. Letter no. 23 02/008, Manson to Ross, 22 August 1895, 70–71.

76. "Reports of Societies: Royal Medical and Churirgical Society (February 11, 1896)," *British Medical Journal*, 15 February 1896: 401–4, quotations on 403 and 404.

77. "Reports of Societies: Royal Medical and Chirurgical Society, (Tuesday, 25 February 1896)," *British Medical Journal*, 29 February 1896, 530–31.

78. Letter no. 29 02/360, Manson to Ross, 21 October 1895, 88, 89.

79. Letter no. 31 02/083, Ross to Manson, 12 December 1895, 91–92.

80. Letter no. 32 02/011, Manson to Ross, 23 December 1895, 92. "I am looking forward to great things from your glycerine mosquitoes. I shall section them first; treat the haemoglobin with weak acetic so as not to dissolve it out, and then stain for the parasite. I believe I shall see the flagellated body in full form, and I believe I shall see flagella on their way to the walls of the mosquito's stomach. Shall I be able to trace them further???? If I can't you must take it up in fresh insects and if you fail with the microscope you must try what experiments will do" (93–94).

81. Letter no. 34 02/012, Manson to Ross, 29 January 1896, 98.

82. Patrick Manson, "The Goulstonian Lectures on the Life-History of the Malaria Germ Outside the Human Body (Lecture I)," *British Medical Journal*, 14 March 1896: 641–46; Lecture II, Ibid., 21 March 1896: 712–17; and Lecture III, 28 March 1896: 774–79.

83. Manson, "The Goulstonian Lectures (Lecture II)," 716.

84. Manson, "The Goulstonian Lectures of (Lecture III)," 777.

85. Ibid. Manson's hopes were steadied—briefly—by the arrival of Ross's consignment of mosquitoes. After examining a single specimen, Manson fired off the following: "Just a line to say EUREKA. That is to say your mosquitoes have turne dout so far to be first rate" (Manson to Ross, Letter no. 39 02/015, 109). Examination of one mosquito, after sectioning and staining, revealed the presence of pigmented spheres and flagella. Manson added a footnote to his published third lecture, informing readers of his intention "ere long to give a more complete description of these and similar preparations." See "The Goulstonian Lectures (Lecture III)," 777. But Manson would have to wait until July 1897, because the quality of the remaining specimens was too poor. "I have had many of your last batch of mosquitoes sectioned, but except in one or two instances, and even in these somewhat doubtfully, have failed to make out the flagella" (see Letter no. 42 02/016, Manson to Ross, 18 April 1896, 113).

86. Amico Bignami, "Hypotheses as to the Life-History of the Malarial Parasite Outside the Human Body (Apropos of an Article by Dr. Patrick Manson)," *Lancet*, 14 November 1896: 1363–67, and 21 November 1896: 1441–44.

87. Ibid., 1443–44. Gordon Harrison has illuminated the differences between Man-

son and Bignami regarding the relationship of the mosquito to malaria disease. "Both accepted the traditional view that the malarial germ belonged by nature in the environment. Bignami was chiefly interested in how it got from the environment into the human blood. Manson was chiefly interested in how it got out and back where it belonged. For Bignami, the mosquito was an inoculating syringe; for Manson she was a pipette and transport system. Neither perceived that her proboscis might be, as in fact it is, a two-way passage, both entrance and exit." Gordon Harrison, *Mosquitoes, Malaria and Man: A History of the Hostilities since 1880* (New York: Dutton, 1978), 59.

88. Bignami cited Laveran's epidemiological inference regarding the coincidence of fever with mosquitoes and its absence with the suppression of mosquitoes; the life-history of filariasis as well as Carlos Finley's assertion that mosquitoes transmitted the cause of yellow fever. "Hypotheses," 1443.

89. Ibid., 1364.

90. Ibid., 1365. Manson did not dispute Bignami's criticism of his a priori reasoning, but remained convinced of the role of the mosquito in the life-history of the *Plasmodium*. Patrick Manson, "Correspondence: Hypotheses as to the Life-History of the Malarial Parasite Outside the Human Body," Ibid., 12 December 1896: 1715–16.

91. Letter No. 48 02/018, Manson to Ross, 12 October 1896, 124.

92. Patrick Manson, "Correspondence: Hypotheses as to the Life-History of the Malarial Parasite Outside the Human Body," Ibid., 12 December 1896: 1715–16.

91. Letter No. 48 02/018, Manson to Ross, 12 Oceober 1896, 124.

92. Patrick Manson, "Correspondence: Hypotheses as to the Life-History of the Malarial Parasite Outside the Human Body," *Lancet*, 12 December 1896: 1715–1716.

93. Ross, *Memoirs*, 179–82, 199. On the position at Agra, see letter no. 38 02/014, Manson to Ross, 18 March 1896, 109.

94. Ross, *Memoirs*, 201–2.

95. Ibid., 202–11.

96. Shortly after Ross reported exflagellation in the spring of 1895, Indian authorities rejected Ross's plan to solicit the financial support of the Maharajah of Patalia for malaria research (Ross, *Memoirs*, 162). Excited by the early progress of the theory, Manson promised to enlist the medical press, Sir Charles Crosthwaite, the permanent undersecretary of state for India, and his patient Anthony MacDonnel, a highly decorated lieutenant-governor of the North West Provinces and Oudh, on Ross's behalf. (See letter no. 16 02/006 Manson to Ross, 45.). "I am preparing a manifesto for the BMA meeting, only some three weeks off, and I think that after this comes out you will be boomed perhaps more than you want. Meanwhile I am intending to interview Hart and perhaps the Lancet people at all events the former, so that he may be up to the ropes and prepared with a stiff leader as soon as the paper is read. I have also some chance of making some influence in your favour at the India Office. I know Charles Crosthwaite and I am sure he will lend a hand if he is approached; I also know Sir MacDonald who I understand is a power in the state. I do not know him well but I see him as a patient, and expect to see him again soon. Him too I shall try to influence" (letter no. 16 02/006, Manson to Ross, 10 July 1895, 45).

97. Letter no. 73 02/114, Ross to Manson, 7 June 1897, 182.

98. Manson to Charles Crosthwaite, 5 July 1897.

99. Ibid.

100. Ernest Hart, "An Address on the Medical Profession in India: Its Position and Its Work," *British Medical Journal*, 29 December 1894, 1469–74. On the reaction, see "Medical Research in India," *British Medical Journal*, 24 August 1895, 488–89, and "Correspondence: The Malarial Parasite," *British Medical Journal*, 19 October 1895, 1001–2.

101. See Douglas M. Haynes, "Social Status and Imperial Service: Tropical Medicine and the British Medical Profession," in David Arnold (ed.), *Warm Climate and Western Medicine: The Emergence of Tropical Medicine* (Amsterdam: Rodopi, 1996), 208–20.

102. Letter no. 83 02/026, Manson to Ross, 8 July 1897, 208–9.

103. Letter no. 90 02/031, Manson to Ross, 11 August 1897, 223.

104. "The Risks of the Study of Malaria," *British Medical Journal*, 17 July 1897, 163.

105. Ross, *Memoirs*, 216. See also letter no. 83 02/026, Manson to Ross, 7 July 1897, 209.

106. Letter no. 84 02/121, Ross to Manson, 27 July 1897, 211.

107. Letter no. 85 02/122, Ross to Manson, 4 August 1897, 214.

108. Letter no. 89 02/124, Ross to Manson, 22 August 1897, 219–22.

109. Letter no. 91 02/125, Ross to Manson, 31 August 1897, 225–27.

110. Letter no. 98 02/034, Manson to Ross, 1 October 1897, 241. Manson hoped "to secure priority for English discovery and partly because it will stimulate others to work on the same lines. It will do you good too by showing that you are not of lying on your oars."

111. Letter No. 105 02/038, Manson to Ross, 17 November 1897, 257.

112. "A Malarial Problem," *British Medical Journal*, 18 December 1897: 1805–6. John Bland-Sutton, a distinguished surgeon and anatomist at Middlesex Hospital who also served as keeper of the animal collection of the Zoological Society, lived across the street from Manson. Manson made the most of this neighbor. Sutton recalled that "when Manson had something unusual, rare, or new, in the way of blood-parasites he would ask me to look at it; he was also keen on the blood-parasites of the animals in the Zoological Gardens." See John Bland-Sutton, *The Story of a Surgeon* (London: Methuen, 1930), 150–52.

113. "A Malarial Problem," 1806.

114. See appendix in Ronald Ross, "On Some Peculiar Pigmented Cells Found in the Mosquito Fed on Malarial Blood," *British Medical Journal*, 18 December 1897, 1787–88.

115. Letter no. 99 02/035, Manson to Ross, 21 October 1897, 242.

116. See appendix, Ross, "On Some Peculiar Pigmented Cells," 1788.

117. Letter no. 94 02/129, Ross to Manson, 27 September 1897, 234–36.

118. Letter no. 95 02/135, Ross to Manson, 28 September 1897, 237.

119. Letter no. 96 02/131, Ross to Manson, 5 October 1897, 238–39; letter no. 97 02/132, Ross to Manson, 12 October 1897, 239–40; letter no. 103 (enclosed with letter no. 106 02/136, 6 December 1897, 251–56). On Rewa post, see Ross, *Memoirs*, 255.

120. Letter no. 103, 255.

121. Letter No. 112 02/039, Manson to Ross, 27 December 1897, 269.

122. Ibid.

122. Ibid.

123. Letter no. 114 02/143, Ross to Manson, 1 February 1898, 275.

124. Ross, *Memoirs*, 259–60.

125. Ibid, 260–67.

126. Letter no. 118 02/147, Ross to Manson, 9 March 1898, 285.

127. Letter no. 117 02/040, Manson to Ross, 7 February 1898, 281–83, and letter no. 119 02/148, Ross to Manson, 15 March 1898, 286–88. The *proteosoma* is one of two blood genera of *Plasmodia sporozoa* that infect birds, the second being *Halteridium*. These parasites not only contain pigment but also replicate asexually within the bloodstream of the bird and sexually in the mosquito.

128. "Report on Meeting of Johns Hopkins Medical Society: On the Pathology of Haematozoan Infections in Birds," *Johns Hopkins Hospital Bulletin* 72 (March 1897): 51–54, and W. G. MacCallum, "On the Haematozoan Infections on Birds," *Johns Hopkins Hospital Bulletin*, 80 (November 1897): 235–36. MacCallam's research appeared in Britain simultaneously. See W. G. MacCallum, "On the Flagellated Form of the Malarial Parasite," *Lancet*, 13 November 1897: 1240–41.

129. Ross, *Memoirs*, 264.

130. Ibid., 267–72.

131. Ibid., 269, 271.

132. Letter no. 125 02/042, Manson to Ross, 9 April 1898, 306.

133. Letter no. 133 02/133, Ross to Manson, 22 June 1898, 327.

134. Ibid. and letter no. 135 02/159, Ross to Manson, 28 June 1898, 331, 332.

135. Letter no. 136 02/160, Ross to Manson, 6 July 1898, 335.

136. Ibid., 336, 337.

137. Letter no. 138 02/161, Ross to Manson, 9 July 1898, 339–43, quotations on p. 340.

138. Letter no. 104 (enclosed with letter no. 105) 02/037, Manson to Ross, 10 November 1897, 256.

139. Letter no. 125 02/042, Manson to Ross, 9 April 1898, 306.

140. Ross, *Memoirs*, 285–87, 317.

141. Gordon Harrison, *Mosquitoes, Malaria, and Man: A History of the Hostilities since 1880* (New York: E. P. Dutton, 1977), 102–8.

142. Letter no. 130, 02/044, Manson to Ross, 29 April 1898, 318–20.

143. Patrick Manson, "The Mosquito-Malaria Theory," *British Medical Journal*, 18 June 1898: 1575–77.

144. Ibid., 1576.

145. Ibid., 1577. Letter No. 137 02/046, Manson to Ross, 24 June 1898, 337–38.

146. Manson, "The Mosquito-Malaria Theory," 1577.

147. Ibid., 1576, 1577. The reference to the " 'divining rod' of preconceived idea" is taken from a review of William Sydney Thayer's *Lectures on the Malarial Fevers* (New York: Appelton, 1897), but the review makes no mention of Manson or his theory. When referring to the growing research literature on malaria, the reviewer noted tartly: "A great deal of valuable material is still mixed, however, with baser mineral, and unfortunately the literature also is encumbered with quantities of spurious ore, consequent mainly upon investigation guided by the 'divining rod' of preconceived idea." See "Notes on New Books: Lectures on the Malarial Fevers," *Johns Hopkins Hospital Bulletin*, December 1897: 266.

148. Manson, "The Mosquito-Malaria Theory," 1576.

149. "Honour to Whom Honour Is Due," *British Medical Journal*, 18 June 1898: 1607–8.

150. Ross, *Memoirs*, 318.

151. Letter no. 139, 02/049, Manson to Ross, 1 July 1898, 344.

152. Letter no. 141 02/050, Manson to Ross, 8 July 1898, 347.

153. Ross, *Memoirs*, 297–305.

154. Letter no. 139 02/049, Manson to Ross, 1 July 1898, 344. Ross was all for it. "The scheme you are going to propose is admirable. No doubt the Government of India will jog up when Chamberlain comes along." Letter no. 138 02/161, Ross to Manson, 9 July 1898, 341.

155. On Manson's illness, see letter no. 137 02/046, Manson to Ross, 24 June 1898, 337; letter no. 139 02/049, Manson to Ross 1 July 1898, 344; and letter no. 143 02/051, Manson to Ross, 15 July 1898, 351.

156. Letter no. 141 02/050, Manson to Ross, 8 July 1898, 347.

157. Letter no. 143 02/051, 351.

158. Letter no. 146 02/052, Manson to Ross, 28 June 1898, 355–56.

159. Patrick Manson, "The Role of the Mosquito in the Evolution of the Malarial Parasite," *Lancet*, 20 August 1898: 488.

160. Ross, *Memoirs*, 306.

161. P. H. Manson-Bahr and Colonel A. Alcock, *The Life and Work of Patrick Manson* (London: Cassell, 1927), 208–20, P. H. Manson-Bahr, *London School of Hygiene and Tropical Medicine, Memoir I: History of the School of Tropical Medicine in London, 1899–1949* (London: H. K. Lewis, 1956), 3–5; P. H. Manson-Bahr, *Patrick Manson: Father of Tropical Medicine* (London: Thomas Nelson & Sons, 1962), 120–28; Robert Kubieck, *The Administration of Imperialism: Joseph Chamberlain at the Colonial Office* (Durham: Duke University Press, 1969), 141–73; Micheal Worboys, "The Emergence of Tropical Medicine: A Study in the Establishment of a Scientific Speciality," in G. Lamaine et al. (eds.), *Perspectives on the Emergence of Scientific Disciplines* (The Hague: Mouton, 1976), 80–87; and John Farley, *Bilharzia: A History of Imperial Tropical Medicine* (Cambridge: Cambridge University Press, 1991), 13–30.

Chapter 5. Domesticating Tropical Medicine

1. I discuss the role of the Colonial Office as employer and source of science funding in "The Social Production of Metropolitan Expertise in Tropical Diseases: The Imperial State, Colonial Service, and the Tropical Diseases Research Fund," *Journal of Science, Technology, and Society* 4, no. 2 (July–December 1999): 4–12.

2. "Medical Appointments in the Colonies," *British Medical Journal*, 4 April 1891, 770.

3. Anne Digby, *Making a Medical Living: Doctors and Patients in the English Market for Medicine, 1720–1911* (Cambridge, England: Cambridge University Press, 1994), 144–147.

4. See James Johnson, *The Influence of Tropical Climates, More Especially of the Climate of India, on European Constitutions; and the Principal Effects and Diseases Thereby Induced, Their Prevention and Removal, and Means of Preserving Health in Hot Climates Rendered Obvious to Europeans of Every Capacity* (London: Thomas and George Greenwood, 1815, 1821); James R. Martin, *The Influence of*

Tropical Climates on European Constitutions, Including Practical Observations on the Nature and Treatment of the Diseases of Europeans on Their Return from Tropical Climates (London: Churchill, 1856, 1861); James Africanus Beale Horton, *The Diseases of Tropical Climates and Their Treatment* (London: Churchill, 1874, 1876); C. S. Grant, *West African Hygiene* (London: E. Stanford, 1884); Fox Tilbury and T. Farquhar, eds., *On Certain Endemic Skin and Other Diseases of India and Hot Climates Generally* (London: J. Churchill, 1876); William Campbell Maclean, *Diseases of Tropical Climates: Lectures Delivered at the Army Medical School* (London: J. Churchill, 1886); Andrew Davidson, ed., *Hygiene and Diseases of Warm Climates* (Edinburgh: Pentland, 1892); and Andrew Davidson, *Geographical Pathology: An Inquiry into the Geographical Distribution of Infective and Climatic Diseases* (Edinburgh: Pentland, 1892).

5. "Medical Appointments in the Colonies," *Lancet*, 21 April 1888, 795.

6. See Ross Palmer, *Simple Directions as to the Treatment of Malarial Fevers, &c* (London: Waterlow, 1897), Public Record Office CO 96/329/196224 [unless otherwise noted, all government documents are from the Public Record Office]; Ross Palmer, *Hints on the Outfit and Preservation of Health on the West Coast of Africa* (Colonial Office Pamphlet, February 1897), and Manson minute and annotation on *Hints on the Outfit and Preservation of Health on the West Coast of Africa* (1 February 1898), CO 96/123/196224.

7. On remuneration, see Digby, *Making a Medical Living*, 135–69.

8. See "Medical Appointments in the Colonies," *British Medical Journal*, 28 August 1897, 558–59.

9. In British Guiana, probationers received £300 with quarters. Thereafter, permanent staff officers received £25 annual increases (with salaries beginning at £400 and topping off at £700). In the Gold Coast colony, an assistant who completed three years of service and "performed his duty in a satisfactory manner and [was] continued in his appointment" received a £20 increase (with salaries beginning at £400 and topping off at £500). "Medical Appointments in the Colonies," *British Medical Journal*, 28 August 1897, 558–59.

10. "Medical Appointments in the Colonies," *British Medical Journal*, 28 August 1897, 558–59; "Medical Appointments in the Colonies," *Lancet*, 21 April 1888: 795.

11. See "Medical Appointments in the Colonies," *Lancet*, 21 April 1888, 795–96.

12. "Correspondence: Colonial Appointments," *British Medical Journal*, 7 February 1880, 231.

13. "Correspondence: Colonial Appointments," *British Medical Journal*, 28 February 1880, 351.

14. Ibid.

15. "Correspondence: Salaries in Ceylon," *British Medical Journal*, 19 June 1880, 958.

16. "Correspondence: Reduction of Salaries in Ceylon," *British Medical Journal*, 4 September 1880, 415.

17. "Correspondence: Registered Practitioner (Grenada)," *British Medical Journal*, 17 July 1880, 114.

18. "Correspondence: Colonial Appointments," *British Medical Journal*, 4 September 1880, 419.

19. "Correspondence: Irregular Practice in the Colonies," *British Medical Journal*, 30 July 1881, 194.

20. "The Colonial Medical Service," *Lancet*, 27 May 1882, 882.

21. "The Colonial Medical Service," *Lancet*, 8 July 1882, 27.

22. "India and the Colonies: West Africa," *British Medical Journal*, 24 May 1884, 1019–20.

23. "The Lancet Commission on Malarial Fever in Tropical Africa," *Lancet*, 2 July 1892, 32.

24. "Ignorance in Tropical Diseases," *British Medical Journal*, 29 December 1894, 1491.

25. "Instruction in Tropical Diseases," *British Medical Journal*, 6 April 1895, 771.

26. No. 13 Middlesex Hospital to CO, 16 March 1898, CO 885/7, 17; No. 14 St. Mary's Hospital to CO, 22 March 1898, CO 885/7, 17–18; No. 18 Charing Cross Hospital, 16 April 1898, CO 885/7, 21; No. 39 Westminister Hospital to CO, 15 July 1898, CO 885/7, 34.

27. See British Parliamentary Papers, *Census of England and Wales* for 1861, General Report 52 (1863), pt. 1, table 1, 247; for 1871, 71 (1873), pt. 2, appendix A, table 107, 113; for 1891, 106 (1893–94), 673; for 1901 CVIII (1904), 92.

28. These data compiled from reports on the Medical Register in the *Lancet*, 14 April 1888, 1:731–32; 26 April 1890, 1:911; 28 March 1891, 723; 2 April 1892, 760; 9 April 1892, 810; 25 March 1893, 661; 17 March 1894, 682; 10 March 1894, 647; 12 January 1895, 109; 16 March 1895, 688; 8 January 1898, 109–10; 2 April 1898, 948; 1 January 1899, 46; 7 January 1899, 46; and 13 May 1899, 1306.

29. For a useful account on state medicine, see Jeanne L. Brand, *Doctors and the State: The British Medical Profession and Government Action in Public Health, 1870-1912* (Baltimore: Johns Hopkins University Press, 1965).

30. Anne Digy, *Making a Medical Living*, 144–47.

31. "Sir Dyce Duckworth: Valedictory Address," *Lancet*, 10 August 1889, 254.

32. "Colonial Medical Appointments," *Lancet*, 11 April 1891, 847.

33. George Evatt, "Notes on the Organisation of the Colonial Medical Service of the Empire," *British Medical Journal*, 26 September 1896, 864.

34. "Correspondence: The Colonial Medical Service," *British Medical Journal*, 14 November 1896, 1479–80.

35. "The Colonial Medical Service: A Rejoinder," *British Medical Journal*, 23 January 1897, 216. This was certainly the sentiment of Herbert J. Read, private secretary to Joseph Chamberlain. Read replied with some peevishness to a resolution from the Committee on "The Organisation of the Colonial Medical Service," which consisted of active and retired imperial doctors as well as civilian practitioners. "These people must be taught the A.B.C. of Colonial Administration. . . . The Cttee [*sic*] think that it is possible to organize one general Colonial Medical Service on the same lines as the AMD or the Indian Medical Service, but the conditions are totally different in the two cases." See Herbert Read, Minute on Letter from Joseph Fayrer and James Cantile, 10 March 1898, Public Record Office CO 323/437/9829, 243–44.

36. Minute on Dr. Charles Gage-Brown's Appointment as Medical Adviser, 2 December 1874, CO 323/318/13769.

37. For Charles Gage-Brown's consultations, see R. R. Bruce of Brighton regarding malarial fever, 6 August 1898, CO 323/439/17888; Tisane Marcellan malarial remedy, CO

323/424/10286; CO 323/472/3166 and 33912. His successor, Patrick Manson, did his share of consultations as well. See "On the Clayton Fire Extinguishing Apparatus," 22 March 1901, CO 323/472/10584, 18 May 1903, CO 323/490/18391 and 24132; On Dr. Theodore Thomson's rat poison, 10 October 1900, CO 323/460/33045; Dr. O'Sullivan *on Black Water Fever in the Colonies, and Protectorates*, CO 323/481/11047; and Sanitary Institute and Principles of Tropical Hygiene, CO 323/490/4560.

38. Dr. John F. Easmon outlined his program in a letter to the Gold Coast governor, William Maxwell. See Easmon to Maxwell, 15 March 1895, CO 96/256/8001, 14–15.

39. This proved to be a contentious problem between Easmon and Maxwell. See Adell Patton Jr., *Physicians, Colonial Racism, and Diaspora in West Africa* (Gainesville: University Press of Florida, 1996), 105–8, 113–22.

40. Gage-Brown to Chamberlain, 25 March 1896, CO 96/285/B6546.

41. Frederic Hodgson to Chamberlain on Training Under Colonial Medical Officer, 22 May 1896, CO 96/273, 3–5.

42. Gage-Brown on Training Under Chief Medical Officer, 2 July 1896, CO 96/273.

43. Minutes on Training Under Chief Medical Officer, 3 August 1896, CO 96/273, 1–2.

44. See Draft Letter from Colonial Office to Governor William Maxwell, 10 February 1897, CO 96/278/24927.

45. On Manson's tenure as medical adviser, see Eli Chernin, "Sir Patrick Manson: Physician to the Colonial Office, 1897–1912," *Medical History* 36, no. 3 (July 1992): 320–30.

46. During his presidential address to the Hong Kong Medical Society, Manson sarcastically volunteered, "The lay mind had abandoned the 'Jos Sedley' and 'Nabob' type but, alas, the profession is for once behind the age—it sticks to its traditions. Anyone who has been through the Suez Canal is assumed in London consulting rooms to have an enlarged or otherwise diseased liver; that he eats and drinks too much, and that he stands in need of blue pills, nitro-nuriatic acid and quinine." Patrick Manson, "Presidential Address," *Transactions of the Hong Kong Medical Society* (1889): 4.

47. Patrick Manson, "The Annual Oration: Malaria and Its Associated Parasite," *Transactions of the Hunterian Society* (1894–95): 21.

48. Letter no. 86 02/028, Manson to Ross, 22 July 1897, in W. F. Bynum and Caroline Overy, eds., *The Beast in the Mosquito: The Correspondence of Ronald Ross and Patrick Manson* (Amsterdam: Rodophi, 1998), 216.

49. According to one account, the introductory address was "valuable in conducing to the punctual attendance of students" and only secondarily in their professional development. Since the subject matter was left to the speaker, it provided him "with an opportunity of delivering his soul upon any subject—even if it be but remotely connected with medicine—to which he may desire to speak." See the *Times* (London), 4 October 1894, 9.

50. Manson boasted to Ronald Ross about his speech. "You will have seen from the medical papers that I have been rubbing it in again about medical education re tropical subjects. That has bruised a good many toes, and has made me enemies as well as many friends. I have only spoken the truth and they can revile as much as they like." Letter no. 99 02/035, Manson to Ross, 21 October 1897, in Bynum and Overy, *The Beast in the Mosquito*, 243.

51. Patrick Manson, "On the Necessity for Special Education in Tropical Medicine," *Lancet*, 2 October 1897, 842–45.

52. See Herbert J. Read, Memorandum on Medical Services, n.d., CO 885/7/26144, 1.

53. Ibid.; Herbert Read to J. Brunton at the War Office, 28 October 1897, CO 147/123, 1–2.

54. H. P. Harvey to Read, 28 October 1897, CO 147/123.

55. See Herbert Read, Memorandum on Medical Services, n.d., CO 885/7/26144, 2.

56. See Minute Book, Seamen's Hospital Society, 13 May 1893, 8 January 1897.

57. Herbert Read to Charles Prescott Lucas on School of Tropical Medicine, 30 November 1898, CO 96/332/27011.

58. See Herbert Read, Memorandum on Medical Services, n.d., CO 885/7/26144, 1–3.

59. No. 17 Seamen's Hospital Society to Colonial Office, 16 April 1898, CO 885/7, 19–20.

60. Robert Kubicek, *The Administration of Imperialism: Joseph Chamberlain at the Colonial Office* (Durham, N.C.: Duke University Press, 1969), 68–91.

61. No. 28 CO to Treasury, 18 June 1898, CO 885/7, 25.

62. No. 29 Treasury to CO, 18 June 1898, CO 885/7, 30.

63. The Federated Malay States and Straits Settlements agreed to contribute £500 jointly (no. 172 Federated Malay States to CO, 23 February 1899 and no. 175 Straits Settlements to CO, 9 February 1899, CO 885/7, 110, 113). The Legislative Council of the Gold Coast voted £1,000 (no. 177 Gold Coast Acting Governor Low to Mr. Chamberlain, 13 February 1899, CO 885/7, 115). Trinidad promised to contribute £750 over two years (Gov. H. E. H. Jerningham to Mr. Chamberlain, 22 February 1899, CO 885/7, 115.) The Lagos Legislative Council voted £1,000 (Gov. Denton to Mr. Chamberlain, 24 February 1899, CO 885/7, 115–16.) The Legislative Council of Hong Kong voted £250 and anticipated a second in the following year (Gov. H. A. Blake to Mr. Chamberlain, 22 February 1899, CO 885/7, 117.) Gambia promised £200 (Gambia Administrator to Mr. Chamberlain, 1 April 1899, CO 885/7, 120.)

64. See enclosure in no. 172 Federated Malay States to CO, 19 February 1899, CO 885/7, 114.

65. No. 205 Gov. A. W. L. Hemming to Mr. Chamberlain, 10 May 1899, CO 885/7, 128.

66. No. 12 CO to General Medical Council, 11 March 1898, CO 885/7, 16.

67. No. 14 St. Mary's Hospital to CO, 22 March 1898, CO 885/7, 17–18; no. 16 St. George's Hospital to CO, 30 March 1898, CO 885/7, 18; no. 18 Charing Cross Hospital to CO, 16 April 1898, CO 885/7, 21–22; no. 44 University College, London to CO, 24 July 1898, CO 885/7, 36; no. 20 University College, Bristol to CO, 30 April 1898, CO 885/7, 22; no. 39 Westminster Hospital to CO, 15 July 1898, CO 885/7, 34; and no. 38 Royal Colleges, Edinburgh to CO, 14 July 1898, CO 885/7, 34.

68. No. 13 Middlesex Hospital to CO, 16 March 1898, CO 885/7, 17; no. 19 Victoria University, Liverpool to CO, 30 April 1898, CO 885/7, 22; no. 26 Yorkshire College, Leeds, to CO, 2 June 1898, CO 885/7, 25; no. 21 Queen's College, Cork, to CO, 2 May 1898, CO 885/7, 21; no. 156 Queen's College, Belfast to CO, 26 January 1899, CO 885/7, 105.

69. No. 22 St. Thomas's Hospital to CO, 9 May 1898, CO 885/7, 22–23.

70. No. 24 St. Bartholomew's Hospital to CO, 1 June 1898, CO 885/7, 24.

71. No. 46 Guy's Hospital to CO, 25 July 1898, CO 885/7, 37.

72. No. 22 St. Thomas's Hospital to CO, 9 May 1898, CO 885/7, 22–23; no. 24 St. Bartholomew's Hospital to CO, 1 June 1898, CO 885/7, 24.

73. "Letter to Editor: Henry C. Burdett," *Times*, 11 July 1898, 12.

74. "Correspondence (John Curnow, John Anderson, and G. R. Turner): A Proposed School for Tropical Medicine," *Lancet*, 23 July 1898, 227.

75. M. Jeanne Peterson, *The Medical Profession in Mid-Victorian London* (Berkeley: University of California Press, 1978), 138–45, 173–88.

76. Ibid. While they accepted the power of the management committee to elect staff, they still thought an appointed subcommittee should have been called together "to give the medical staff the opportunity of discussing the qualifications of candidates for the appointment of Surgeon to the Branch Hospital and reporting to the Committee, notwithstanding that as there were only two candidates both names must be submitted to the Committee." Minute book, Seamen's Hospital Society, 27 March 1896. See also "Medical Officers and Hospital Governors," *Lancet*, 16 August 1856, 203–4.

77. P. Michelli, secretary of the Seamen's Hospital Society, to Charles Prescott Lucas, undersecretary of state of CO (in file on School of Tropical Medicine), 30 November 1898, CO 96/332, 2–3.

78. On Manson's self-misrepresentations, see "Correspondence: The Seamen's Hospital Society and the Visiting Staff," *Lancet*, 24 December 1898, 1737. On the diagnosis of tropical disease cases, see "Correspondence (Dr. Curnow)," *Lancet*, 30 October 1897, 1143.

79. Anderson taught tropical medicine at St. Mary's Hospital and used the clinical cases at the Dreadnought for teaching purposes. See Anderson's letter in enclosure in no. 14 St. Mary's Hospital to CO, 2 March 1898, CO 885/7, 17–18. Curnow also taught tropical medicine at King's College, University of London, no. 105 King's College to C.O., 22 November 1898, CO 885/7, 69–70.

80. "Annotations: The Teaching of Tropical Diseases in London," *Lancet*, 16 July 1898: 158; "The Proposed School of Tropical Medicine (Senior Visiting Physician)," *Daily Chronicle*, 26 November 1898, 6; and "Correspondence (John Curnow): The Proposed School of Tropical Medicine," *Lancet*, 17 December 1898, 1661.

81. "Medical News: General Medical Council," ibid, 26 November 1898: 1448.

82. No. 189 Andrew Davidson to CO, 25 April 1898, CO 885/7, 121.

83. "The Teaching of Tropical Diseases in London," *Lancet*, 16 July 1898, 158.

84. "Correspondence: The Proposed School of Tropical Medicine," *Lancet*, 17 December 1898, 1654.

85. "Instruction in Tropical Medicine," *Lancet*, 10 December 1898, 1579.

86. "Correspondence (John Curnow, John Anderson, and G. R. Turner): The Seamen's Hospital Society and Its Visiting Staff," *Lancet*, 24 December 1898, 1737.

87. William Broadbent to Chamberlain, n.d., CO 96/322/28213, 3–4.

88. A. E. Collins to Charles Prescott Lucas, undersecretary of state, n.d., CO 94/322/MO 28213.

89. Charles Prescott Lucas's Minute on Sir William Broadbent, 6 December 1898, CO 96/332.

90. "The Proposed School of Tropical Medicine," *British Medical Journal*, 17 December 1898, 1654–55. Manson reversed himself on a conference with Broadbent. See Collins to Chamberlain on Broadbent conference, 10 December 1898, CO 96/332.

91. " 'Dreadnought' Hospital, Greenwich and Its Visiting Medical Staff," *Lancet*, 1 April 1899: 909.

92. See entry for Alfred Jones in *Dictionary of National Biography, 2d Supplement, 1901–11* (Oxford: Oxford University Press, 1912), 379–80.

93. Alfred Jones to CO, 11 November 1898 and 17 November, CO 96/285. Of Jones's offer, one imperial official noted in a minute: "It is curious that good men like Al. Jones should be taken in by such rubbish as Dr. Hayward appears to have talked." Memorandum on Malarial Fever: Homeopathic Treatment, 17 November 1898, CO 96/285.

94. "Schools of Tropical Medicine in Liverpool and Elsewhere," *Lancet*, 21 January 1899, 181–82.

95. Alfred Jones to CO, 6 January 1899, CO 995/7.

96. Charles Prescott Lucas to Chamberlain on Liverpool recognition, 17 January 1899, CO 96/353, 3–5.

97. No. 159 CO to A. Jones, 1 February 1899, CO 885/7. See also minutes to Lucas on Jones' response to Chamberlain, CO 96/353, 1.

98. A. Jones to C.O., 11 February 1899, CO 96/353, 1.

99. No. 171 CO to Jones, 23 February 1899, CO 96/353.

100. Miscellaneous no. 143 memorandum respecting proposed government assistance to the London School of Tropical Medicine, n.d., CO 887/8, 1.

101. No. 225 CO To SHS, 30 June 1899, CO 885/7, 141; no. 1 SHS to CO, 27 November 1900, CO 885/7, 1; and no. 71 CO to SHS, 18 September 1900, CO 885/7, 38.

102. Miscellaneous no. 143 memorandum respecting proposed government assistance to the London School of Tropical Medicine, n.d., CO 887/8, 3–5.

Chapter 6. The Tropical Diseases Research Fund and Specialist Science at the London School of Tropical Medicine

1. On the medical adviser position, see "Minute on Appointment of Dr. Charles Gage-Brown," 30 November 1874, Public Record Office CO 323/318/13769, 279–81, and "Minute on Appointment of Dr. Patrick Manson," March 1897, Public Record Office CO 323/424/4610. Unless otherwise noted, all government records are from the Public Record Office.

2. On the relationship between the Local Government Board and the Colonial Office, see letter from W. H. Power of the Local Government on Yellow Fever and the Panama Canal, 16 December 1902, CO 323/477/52829, 664–65, and Minute on Powers, CO 323/477/6889, 148–51.

3. See "Medical Appointments in the Colonies," *Lancet*, 21 April 1888, 795–96.

4. Several recent studies emphasize the benefit of Western medicine to the empire over time. See Philip Curtin, *Death by Migration: Europe's Encounter with the Tropical World in the Nineteenth Century* (Cambridge: Cambridge University Press, 1989); David Arnold, *Colonizing the Body* (Berkeley: University of California Press, 1993); and Mark Harrison, *Public Health in British India: Anglo-Indian Preventive Medicine, 1859–1914* (Cambridge: Cambridge University Press, 1994).

5. For representative ordinances and reports, see British Parliamentary Papers, *Reports from Colonies for 1883* (45, 1886), no. 1 Mauritius (Seychelles and Rodrigues), 8; no. 4 Gambia, 124; no. 13 Falkland Islands, 198–99, no. 14 Malta, 204–5, 211; and no. 16 Gibraltar, 223–24; *Reports from Colonies for 1893* (56, 1894); no. 107 Hong Kong, 103; no. 114 Malta, 193; and *Plague Report for Hong Kong for 1895* (57, 1896), 617–25.

6. On the marginal role of medical personnel in the empire, see Douglas M. Haynes,

"Social Status and Imperial Service: Tropical Medicine and the British Medical Profession in the Nineteenth Century," in David Arnold (ed.), *Warm Climates and Western Medicine: The Emergence of Tropical Medicine, 1500–1900* (Amsterdam: Rodopi, 1996), 217–19. Both Arnold and Harrison show how the fiscal and political concerns of the government of India checked the spread of preventive medicine. See David Arnold, *Colonizing the Body* (Berkeley: University of California Press, 1993), and Harrison, *Public Health in British India*.

7. The coverage of the secondary literature on public health policy in the empire is limited but informative. On Africa, see Raymond E. Dumett, "The Campaign Against Malaria and the Expansion of Scientific Medical and Sanitary Services in British West Africa, 1899–1910," *African Historical Studies* 12 (1968): 153–95; Thomas Gale, "Segregation in British West Africa," *Cahiers d'etudes africaines* 80 (1980): 495–506; and Thomas Gale, "The Struggle Against Disease in Sierra Leone: Early Sanitary Reforms in Freetown," *Africana Research Bulletin* (Freetown) 6, no. 2 (1976): 29–44; Maynard Sawnson, " 'The Sanitation Syndrome': Bubonic Plague and Urban Native Policy in Cape Colony, 1900–1909," *Journal of African History* 18, no. 3 (1977): 387–410; John Cell, "Anglo-Indian Medical Theory and the Origins of Segregation in West Africa," *American Historical Review* 91 (1986): 307–35. For Asia and the Pacific, see Donald Denoon, *Public Health in Papua New Guinea: Medical Possibility and Social Constraint, 1884–1984* (Cambridge: Cambridge University Press, 1989); G. B. Endacott, *A History of Hong Kong* (Oxford: Oxford University Press, 1958), 96–97, 114–16, 183–88, 199–203, 216–20, and 278–79; and Mary Sutpen, "Not What, but Where: Bubonic Plague and the Reception of Germ Theories in Hong Kong and Calcutta, 1894–1897," *Journal of the History of Medicine* 52 (January 1997): 81–113. For a related study, see Kerrie L. MacPherson, *A Wilderness of Marshes: The Origins of Public Health in Shanghai, 1843–1893* (Hong Kong: Oxford University Press, 1987); and Alan Mayne, " 'The Dreadful Scourge': Responses to Smallpox in Sydney and Melbourne, 1881–2," in Roy MacLeod and Milton Lewis (eds.), *Disease, Medicine, and Empire* (London: Routledge, 1988), 219–37.

8. See Clement Francis Goodfellow, *Great Britain and South African Confederation, 1870–1881* (Cape Town: Oxford University Press, 1966).

9. John S. Galbraith, *MacKinnon and East Africa* (Cambridge: Cambridge University Press, 1972).

10. Quoted in Peter Alter, *The Reluctant Patron: Science and the State in Britain, 1850–1920*, trans. Angela Davies (New York: Oxford University Press, 1987), 19.

11. Roy MacLeod, "The Royal Society and the Government Grant: Notes on the Administration of Scientific Research, 1849–1914," *Historical Journal* 14, no. 2 (1971): 325–26, 329–33. In reversing the recommendation of the Treasury, the Society received permission to reserve any surplus rather than restoring it.

12. Ibid., 336–48.

13. See MacLeod, "The Royal Society and the Government Grant," 323–58. For an informative survey on support for British science, see Alter, *The Reluctant Patron*, 13–74, 138–89.

14. Royal Society, Council minutes, item 7, 310.

15. Paul Cranefield, *Science and Empire: East Coast Fever in Rhodesia and Transvaal* (Cambridge: Cambridge University Press, 1991), 330–31.

16. J. N. P. Davies, "The Cause of Sleeping Sickness? Entebbe 1902–1903," *East African Medical Journal* 39, no. 3 (March 1962): 81–98.

17. The governor of Natal and Zululand, Sir Walter Hely-Hutchinson, specifically requested Bruce. When Hely-Hutchinson was lieutenant governor of Malta, Bruce in 1884 identified the cause of Malta fever (*Micrococcus melitensis*). See Col. E. E. Vella, "Major-General Sir David Bruce," *Journal of the Royal Army Medical Corps* 119, no. 3 (July 1973): 132–35.

18. No. 66 British Guiana Governor Sir W. J. Sendall to Mr. Chamberlain, September 1898, CO 885/7, 50. For the original request, see no. 58, Mr. Chamberlain to Governor Sir W. J. Sendall, September 1898, CO 885/7, 47. The conditions of Daniels's participation were generous. During his absence, he received his £450 salary and drew vacation leave and half-pay for the remainder, and the period away was to be counted toward his seniority and pension. Although Chamberlain regarded the payment of half-pay and the guarantee as the contribution of the colony toward the malaria expedition, he reserved the right to solicit additional contributions for imperial initiatives.

19. For the requests, see no. 96 CO to Crown Agents, 9 November 1898, CO 885/7, 64–65, and no. 111 CO to the Governors of Gambia, Sierra Leone, Lagos, and the Gold Coast, 25 November 1898, CO 885/7, 77–78. For the terms of the salaries of the commissioners, see no. 101 to CO Mr. J. W. W. Stephens and Mr. S. R. Christophers, 19 November 1898, CO 885/7, 66–67.

20. Royal Society, Council minutes, item 7, 310; letter from the Treasury cited in Davies, "The Cause of Sleeping Sickness? 88.

21. Lt. Gen. Sir William MacArthur, "An Account of Some of Sir David Bruce's Researches, Based on His Own Manuscript Notes," *Transactions of the Royal Society of Tropical Medicine and Hygiene* 49, no. 5 (September 1955): 410.

22. Patrick Manson to Herbert Read, 9 August 1898, CO 96/327/17923; and Manson to Lucas, 21 August 1898, CO 96/327/19030.

23. Royal Society to CO, 2 August 1898, CO 885/7/17424.

24. Royal Society to CO, 16 August 1898, CO 885/7/18431.

25. See *A Short Account of the Craggs Prize, 1899-1911* (London: London School of Tropical Medicine, 1912), 1–2.

26. Miscellaneous no. 143 memorandum regarding proposed government assistance for the London School of Tropical Medicine, n.d., CO 887/8, 6. The Colonial Office also offered the medical services of the London School to colonial personnel—for a fee. For personnel who received £400 or less, hospital charges ranged from one to two guineas per day. But it is unlikely that this service generated much revenue. See no. 1 Seamen's Hospital Society to CO, 27 November 1899, CO 885/7, 1.

27. For authorization of Manson's request, see no. 18 CO, 5 March 1900, CO 885/7, 9–10.

28. On London School personnel, see L. W. Sambon to CO, 5 August 1900, CO 885/7/27112; "Obituary: The Late Patrick Thurburn Manson," *Journal of Tropical Medicine*, 1 April 1901, 110; and "Correspondence (D. C. Rees): Experimental Proof of the Malaria-Mosquito Theory," *British Medical Journal*, 6 October 1900, 1054–55.

29. Private donations financed the expedition. Miscellaneous no. 143 memorandum regarding proposed government assistance to the London School of Tropical Medicine, CO 887/8, 8. The Christmas Island Phosphate Company also contributed to the endeavor, though not always reliably. See letter from H. E. Durham, February 1902, to P. Michelli, London School of Tropical Medicine records, truck #1, Seamen's Hospital Society, Greenwich.

30. Davies, "The Cause of Sleeping Sickness?" 81–98.

31. On remuneration, see Ronald Ross's report to the Tropical Diseases Advisory Board on the need to lengthen the duration of the tropical disease course from two to three months. Ronald Ross Archives, School of Hygiene and Tropical Medicine, University of London.

32. On the school's personnel, see *The London School of Tropical Medicine, Sessions, 1899–1900* (London: E. G. Berryman, 1899), 25–26.

33. Ibid., 4–5, 10–24.

34. Ibid., 27.

35. In 1899 and 1900, fifty-four and seventy-four students, respectively, completed the courses. See *A Short History of the Craggs Prize, 1899–1911* (London School of Tropical Medicine, 1912), 5.

36. Miscellaneous no. 143 memorandum regarding proposed government assistance to the London School of Tropical Medicine, CO 887/8, 5–6.

37. Ibid., 5–6, 8, 11–13.

38. Ibid., 11–13.

39. On Chamberlain's circular, see no. 1 Colonial Office to Sir J. West Ridgeway, Sir Patrick Manson, Sir R. Moor, and Sir T. Barlow, 173 miscellaneous correspondence in connection with the Advisory Board of the Tropical Diseases Research Fund, no. 1 CO 885/9.

40. Enclosure of Dr. William Prout to Colonial Secretary, 10 September 1899, in no. 258 Acting Governor of Sierra Leone Nathan to Chamberlain, September 1899, CO 885/7.

41. Ibid.

42. No. 258 Acting Governor Nathan to Chamberlain, 30 September 1899, and no. 13 Malaria Investigation Committee to CO, 27 February 1900, CO 885/7.

43. Enclosure by Charles Wilberforce Daniels, 30 July 1903, on Education in, and Investigation of, Tropical Diseases, in no. 104 Federated Malay States High Commissioner Sir F. A. Sweetenham to Chamberlain, 12 September 1903, CO 885/7.

44. Ibid. Major Will, principal medical officer of the East African and Uganda Protectorates, endorsed Daniels's proposal for regional laboratories while suggesting the Entebbe Laboratory as a candidate for East Africa. Although Will believed that the financial position of the protectorate prevented relieving medical officers of all other work for work in the laboratory, he concurred that specialized training in the periphery was preferable. "It is, whether better results than are at present obtained would not be secured by medical officers on first appointment receiving their instruction in tropical diseases at such an institute or laboratory, instead of, as at present at a school of tropical medicine in England. In the former, material for practical work would always be abundant, whereas in the latter, although theoretical teaching may be excellent, there must necessarily at times be a paucity of material for practical instruction." No. 22 FO to CO, 15 February 1904, CO 885/9, 14.

45. Sir Michael Foster to Charles Prescott Lucas, 7 August 1900, CO 267/471.

46. On the inadequate funding for laboratory science in physiology, see Gerald Geison, *Michael Foster and the Rise of the Cambridge School of Physiology: The Scientific Enterprise in Late Victorian Society* (Princeton: Princeton University Press, 1978), 41–42, 130–31. On the amateur tradition in geology, see Roy Porter, "Gentlemen

and Geology: The Emergence of a Scientific Career, 1660–1920," *Historical Journal* 21, no. 4 (1978): 809–36.

47. The endowment of medicine and science in general was a constant refrain. See "The Month: Sir Michael Foster" and "Science Blatant," *Practitioner*, March 1900, 244–45; "The Month: The Endowment of Medicine," "Laboratories Past and Present," "Medicine Not Mendicant," "The Duty of Millionaires Towards Medicine," *Practitioner*, July 1900, 2–7.

48. Sir Michael Foster to Sir M. Ommanney and Chamberlain, 5 August 1900, CO 267/471.

49. Sir Michael Foster to Charles Prescott Lucas, 7 August 1900, CO 267/471.

50. Chamberlain to Charles Prescott Lucas on Foster, 6 August 1900, CO 267/471.

51. In reply to a request from a deputation of representatives of various chambers of commerce, which included Ross, for a sanitary commission in West Africa, Chamberlain made his opinion clear about experts: They were incapable of balancing the needs of public health with the inelasticity of the public exchequer. "Whatever commission went to those colonies for this purpose must bear in mind what was practical as well as what was ideally desirable. It was quite clear that it must give weighty consideration to the question of cost unless they were to get into financial trouble, which would be more serious than anything else. If the Government sent out a purely scientific expedition they would be handing over practically the decision about the cost, which was really a point for laymen. The experts were not qualified, whatever their scientific acquirements might be with regard to the treatment of disease, to undertake full consideration of the financial aspect of the situation, and no cooperation in this country would consent to put its finances in the hands of a sanitary commissioner, however eminent he might be." *Times*, 16 March 1901, 9. For the public fallout that followed Ross's privately financed control experiment in Sierra Leone, see "Minute on Royal Society," July–August 1903, CO 261/471.

52. No. 1 CO to Sir West Ridgeway et al. on Advisory Board of the Tropical Diseases Research Fund, CO 885/9.

53. See enclosure in no. 3 Australia Mr. Lyttelton to Governor Sir G. R. Le Hunt, 31 August 1904, CO 885/9, 4–5; and "Sources of Promised Funds" table in minutes of first meeting of the Advisory Board, 1 November 1904, CO 885/9, 8.

54. Chamberlain resigned over imperial tariff policy in 1903. See Peter T. Marsh, *Joseph Chamberlain, Entrepreneur in Politics* (New Haven: Yale University Press, 1994), 558–80.

55. No. 1 CO to Sir West Ridgeway et al. on the Advisory Board of the Tropical Diseases Research Fund, 8 July 1904, CO 885/9.

56. For Manson's proposal, see appendix in no. 4 minutes of first meeting of the Advisory Board of the Tropical Diseases Research Fund, 1 November 1904, 6–8, CO 885/9, Miscellaneous no. 173 correspondence [July 1904–December 1906] in connection with the Advisory Board for the Tropical Diseases Research Fund. P. Michelli, secretary to the SHS, specified in a letter to Read how the London School intended to use the positions: "That the tutor or director shall allot their respective teaching work to the demonstrator, the protozoologist and the helmintholgist, and himself, besides exercising a general supervision of the School, shall teach in the laboratory for a certain number of hours each day, and be convenient for reference in other times. . . . The protozoologist to teach in the general laboratory the methods for finding and studying protozoa, say for one hour

a day for a certain number of days each session; to be ready to teach higher protozoology in his own laboratory; to work out any current protozoological problems, and to advance the science, especially in its bearing on tropical medicine. . . . The helminthologist to do similar work in his own subject. The lecturers to spare the students details of the natural history such as can be better taught to students in the laboratories by the special teachers, confining themselves as far as possible to more purely medical matters." CO 885/9, no. 12, SHS to CO, 12 November 1904, 13–15. Miscellaneous No. 173. Correspondence [July 1904–December 1906] in connection with the Advisory Board for the Tropical Disease Research Fund.

57. Ibid, 6.

58. Ibid, 7.

59. See no. 4 minutes of the first meeting of the Advisory Board, 1 November 1904, 6–10; Michael Foster, "Scientific Uses of Hospitals," *Nineteenth Century*, January 1901, 57–63, and "Should the University of London Include Polytechnics?" *Nineteenth Century*, October 1901, 675–82.

60. No. 4 minutes of the first meeting of the Advisory Board, 1 November 1904, 6–7.

61. Ibid., 9.

62. Ibid., 6.

63. No. 13 minutes of second meeting of the Advisory Board of the Tropical Diseases Research Fund, 15 November 1904, 15.

64. This was not the first time. In 1899, Manson sought the support of Chamberlain when SHS contemplated affiliating with the faculty of medicine of the University of London. Manson feared that the two-month course was too short to satisfy university authorities. "Could Mr. Chamberlain work this for us?" he wrote to Lucas. "Needless to say should we get this the advantages will not be altogether on the side of the school but it would exercise our . . . influence to the benefit of the London University." Manson to Lucas on the University of London, 4 December 1899, CO 96/350/33838. Lucas was noncommittal, and the SHS decided not to take any further action on the matter. Lucas on Manson, 5 December 1899, CO 96/350/33838.

65. No. 13 minutes of second meeting of the Advisory Board of the Tropical Diseases Research Fund, 15, 16.

66. No. 4 minutes of first meeting of the Advisory Board of the Tropical Diseases Research Fund, 9–10.

67. Ibid, 6–7, 9–10. The board also authorized £500 for the helminthology position for five years. No. 6 CO to SHS, 4 November 1904, CO 885/9.

68. SHS to CO, 12 November 1904, CO 885/9.

69. No. 119 CO to FO and India Office, 30 November 1903, CO 885/7.

70. No. 13 minutes of second meeting of the Advisory Board of the Tropical Diseases Research Fund, 15–16.

71. Minutes of the third meeting of the Advisory Board of the Tropical Diseases Research Fund, 13 December 1904, 22–25.

72. Ibid., 22–23.

73. Manson to Read, October 1906, CO 323/524/37292.

74. Ibid.

75. Read on the entomology request, 11 October 1906, CO 323/524/37292.

76. Ibid.

77. Minutes of the second meeting of the Advisory Board of the Tropical Diseases Research Fund, 27 November 1906, CO 885/9, 82–83.

78. Ibid, 82.

79. No. 55 Treasury to CO, 27 August 1907, 38–39 CO 885/18; and minutes of the advisory committee of the Tropical Diseases Research Fund, 30 May 1907, 27, CO 885/18.

80. See British Parliamentary Papers, "Report of the Advisory Committee of the Tropical Diseases Research Fund for 1906" (68, 1907), 4; and British Parliamentary Papers, "Report of the Advisory Committee of the Tropical Diseases Research Fund for 1909" (71, 1908), 4.

81. Item 6, minutes of the first ordinary meeting of the Tropical Diseases Research Fund Advisory Committee, 30 May 1907, CO 855/18, 27; and British Parliamentary Papers, "Report of the Advisory Committee for 1909" (66, 1910), 2. On the creation of the Cambridge Professorship, see British Parliamentary Papers, "Report of the Advisory Committee of the Tropical Diseases Research Fund for 1906" (68, 1907), 643.

82. Manson to Herbert Read, 12 February 1912, CO 323/605/25736.

83. Patrick Manson to P. H. Manson-Bahr, 10 January 1919, no. 13, Research Correspondence, F. 24–34. Contemporary Medical Archives, Wellcome Institute for the History of Medicine.

84. P. H. Manson-Bahr, *Patrick Manson: The Father of Tropical Medicine* (London: Nelson and Sons, 1962), 129–36.

85. Ibid., 144–45.

86. Ibid.

87. "Speech Before the General Supporters of the London School of Tropical Medicine," circa 1911, Wellcome Tropical Institute/Royal Society of Tropical Medicine, Contemporary Medical Archives, Wellcome Institute for the History of Medicine, F. 50.

Epilogue: From White Man's Burden to White Man's Grave

1. Sir George McRobert, "Presidential Address: Empire into Commonwealth," *Transactions of the Royal Society of Hygiene and Tropical Medicine* 55, no. 5 (1961): 492.

2. Kevin M. De Cock, Sebastian B. Lucas, David Mabey, and Eldryd Parry, "Tropical Medicine for the Twenty-first Century," *British Medical Journal* 311 (1995): 860.

3. "Will Tropical Medicine Move to the Tropics?" *Lancet*, 347 (1996): 629.

4. D. J. Weatherall, "Tropical Medicine in and Out of the Tropics," *Lancet* 347 (1996): 1111.

5. Ibid. For the death of Caroline Fraser, see "Malaria Victim Had Failed to Complete Course of Tablets," *Times* (London), 10 May 1996, 5.

Index

Acknowledgments

In researching and writing this book, I have benefited from the intellectual labor of scholars, the expertise and financial support of several institutions, and the encouragement of friends and family. Thomas Laqueur and Thomas Metcalf have been generous with their time and advice. I also would like to thank William Bynum and Roy Porter, who assisted me during my research in London. Peter Hoffenburg of the University of Hawaii and my UC Irvine colleagues Karl Hufbauer, Robert Moeller, and Daniel Schroeter read drafts of the manuscript and always provided constructive criticism for which I am immensely grateful. As research assistants, David Johnson and Sharlene Sayegh were generous with their time, uncommonly resourceful, and always supportive.

Without the expertise of numerous librarians and archivists, this project would have been stillborn. I therefore want to thank the staffs at the University of Aberdeen, the Seamen's Hospital Society, the Wellcome Institute for the History of Medicine, where the Manson Papers are housed; Mary Gibson, Ronald Ross Papers archivist of the School of Hygiene and Tropical Medicine, the University of London; the Public Record Office at Kew; the British Library; the Royal College of Physicians; the United States Library of Medicine; and the interlibrary loan department of the University of California, Irvine, for their collective patience and diligence on my behalf. The financial assistance and resources of the Department of History of the University of California, the Fulbright Foundation, the University of California President's Postdoctoral Program, and the UC Irvine School of the Humanities together enabled me to visit archives in England and Scotland and afforded me time to write. All of this effort would have come to naught without the support of a capable editor. It has been my distinct pleasure to work with Patricia Smith at the University of Pennsylvania Press. Of course, books are not written by families, but it would have been impossible for me to complete this one without the unconditional love of my mother and father, seven brothers and sister, and the sustaining intellectual collaboration and emotional support of my stunning spouse, Katrinka.